An Ethics Casebook for Hospitals
Practical Approaches to Everyday Cases

An Ethics Casebook for Hospitals
Practical Approaches to Everyday Cases

Mark G. Kuczewski
Rosa Lynn B. Pinkus

GEORGETOWN UNIVERSITY PRESS / WASHINGTON, D.C.

Georgetown University Press, Washington, D.C.
© 1999 by Georgetown University Press. All rights reserved.
Printed in the United States of America

10   9   8   7   6   5   4   3   2

THIS VOLUME IS PRINTED ON ACID-FREE OFFSET BOOK PAPER

Library of Congress Cataloging-in-Publication Data

An ethics casebook for hospitals : practical approaches to everyday
   cases / Mark G. Kuczewski, Rosa Lynn B. Pinkus.
     p.   cm.
   Includes bibliographical references and index.
   ISBN 0-87840-723-5 (pbk.)
    1. Medical ethics—Case studies.   2. Hospital care—Moral and
ethical aspects—Case studies.   3. Medical ethics committees.
I. Kuczewski, Mark G.   II. Pinkus, Rosa Lynn B.
R725.5.E88   1999
174'.2—dc21   98-44652

Contents

Section Four. The Family in Medical Decision Making   99

Section Five. Organizational and Institutional Ethics   123

Section Six. Rehabilitation Ethics   141

Section Seven. Professional Responsibility: Employers, Colleagues, and Others   161

Section Eight. AIDS: Problems of Confidentiality   179

Preface

WHAT IS DIFFERENT ABOUT THIS CASEBOOK?

This book is a collection of cases with commentary and bibliographic resources designed especially for educational efforts in hospitals. Most of the cases were submitted from hospitals not affiliated with an academic health science center. They reflect the day-to-day moral struggles within the walls of hospitals typically described as community hospitals. While most of the hospitals were labeled "community," they vary greatly. Some are rural, others suburban, and a number are situated in urban settings. Bed capacity ranges from 40 to 400; some were tertiary care facilities; some had mature ethics committees while others were struggling to develop an ethics mechanism. Nonetheless, one common element was that "research" was not a major emphasis nor was the teaching of residents usually a priority. As a result, the cases are not the esoteric high-tech dilemmas of the academic medical center but deal with fundamental problems that are pervasive in health-care delivery in the United States.

Instead of focusing on esoteric procedures such as organ transplantation, genetic engineering, or experimental protocols, this casebook deals with problems such as where to send a frail elderly patient who no longer seems able to care for herself but refuses to go to a nursing home, determining whether a patient has the mental capacity to make his own decisions regarding his treatment, what role the family should play in making a treatment decision when the choice made would greatly affect them, what a family should do when they suspect that their mother is not getting proper care, and what a hospital should do when it is getting "stuck" with too many unpaid bills. This kind of problem is the "stuff" of clinical ethics across most of the country, but only rarely does it provide the focus for ethics casebooks.

Given the recent changes in health-care delivery, it is no longer as useful to distinguish the lines between the community hospital and the academic medical center. During the years since the first few cases of the casebook were compiled, six of the contributing hospitals have either been purchased by or have formed a formal affiliation with a new integrated health-care system that has as its focus the academic teaching hospital. Thus, what was originally "outside the walls" of the academic health center is now inside or at least passes more fluidly between the institutions.

What is most notable about our range of cases is that they include the basic issues articulated since the birth of our discipline of biomedical ethics. The context of health-care delivery has evolved but the basic problems of truth-telling, informed consent, assessing decision-making capacity, and end-of-life decisions remain. Health-care professionals in all hospital settings are being confronted with these common dilemmas and must rely upon a common frame of reference. Hence the title *An Ethics Casebook for Hospitals: Practical Approaches to Everyday Cases.*

The astute reader of these cases will also notice another intriguing feature of the book. The cases presented here come with a variety of problems that cannot be neatly categorized. For easy reference, we have separated the cases according to topical sections such as "Consent and Competence," "Discharge Dilemmas," and "The Family in Medical Decision Making." But the cases in these sections usually exhibit a great deal of overlap, and many could be reassigned to another section. That is, problems concerning where to place patients involve families, problems that involve the wishes of family members may require assessments of the patient's decision-making capacity, etc. As a result, these cases provide the opportunity to sort through the many layers and dimensions of clinical experience and thematize elements of the case that the commentators may have ignored.

The cases are ideal for use by hospital ethics committees and any health-care professional who is undertaking responsibilities as a peer educator in clinical medical ethics. Such people may have some ethics training from participating in a graduate bioethics program, an intensive bioethics course, or a regional network of health-care ethics committees (HEC). These newly trained ethics resource persons are often asked to design or provide continuing medical education in clinical ethics for their colleagues. Such educational efforts may take the form of case conferences or "ethics rounds" at the ethics committee meeting. A problematic case is provided for discussion, and the ethical issues involved are fleshed out. Real-life cases provide the best material for these gatherings. Such cases are pertinent to the experiences of the hospital staff, and their unique features reflect the depth and intricacy of conflict resolution in a way that few creative writers of fiction could imitate. This book was developed to provide easy access to a range of cases and supporting materials for such teaching. Similarly, this text will be useful in college and graduate school courses in biomedical ethics or health policy. Instructors who desire "thick description" of the context of ethical questions will find this book of interest.

This casebook reflects a health-care environment in transition. Its strength is that it provides lessons for a community of health-care providers and users. We hope that it takes a small step forward in communicating the concerns, dilemmas, and resolutions to thorny ethical problems faced by today's health-care professionals.

HOW WAS THE CASEBOOK DEVELOPED?

This book is a collection of cases, most of which were submitted by representatives of the hospitals participating in the Consortium Ethics Program (CEP).[1] The CEP is the regional ethics network of western Pennsylvania.[2] This program helps health-care institutions in the western Pennsylvania region meet their ethics needs by training two representatives from each hospital in medical ethics and assisting them in the design and implementation of an institutional ethics plan. As a training and educational exercise, the participants were asked to identify a case in their hospital that raised ethical questions. Over an extended period of time, the hospital representatives and CEP faculty Mark Kuczewski and Rosa Lynn Pinkus refined these presentations into the material included in this book. Mark Kuczewski and Rosa Lynn Pinkus take full responsibility for the content of this text.

WHAT FEATURES ARE INCLUDED IN THE CASEBOOK?

(a) **Key Terms and Bibliography** Anyone who leads a case discussion in ethics for the first time feels a certain apprehension. Because a working acquaintance with recent developments and trends in the literature can dramatically reduce this anxiety, reading an article or two that has been well received is usually the best medicine. So, we have included both relevant citations at the end of each case and a user-friendly bibliography at the back of the casebook. These citations are in no way meant to be exhaustive. However, they provide reference to material and arguments that are usually considered representative of the mainstream. As a result, we have given priority to "classic" works in the field such as those by the President's Commission for the Study

---

1. As this project gained momentum, four cases from volunteers around the country were also submitted and add greatly to the richness of the book. Two cases were written under the sponsorship of a grant from the Jewish Health-care Foundation and appear in "AIDS and the Community" (an unpublished casebook).

2. The CEP is a collaborative project of the Center for Medical Ethics of the University of Pittsburgh and the Hospital Council of Western Pennsylvania and its 38 institutional members.

of Ethical Problems in Medicine and Biomedical and Behavioral Research and related scholarship.

Each case is preceded by one or more key terms. These are words that are commonly used in discussing the types of issues evidenced in the case. For instance, a case in which full information is not provided to a patient may be preceded by the key terms: Informed Consent, Truth-Telling. Reference to key articles from the list is made in the "Commentary" section that follows the case.

Our bibliographic references should, however, be seen as only a beginning. The key terms can also be used as a starting point to search any medical library and procure a wealth of additional quality information. The inquisitive user of this book will want to become familiar with some of the common databases such as Medline and Bioethicsline (also available by calling 1-800-MED-ETHX) on which these descriptive terms can be run.

(b) The Cases   These real-life cases have been altered to protect confidentiality. A number of headings follow the telling of the story of each case. We provide sections that highlight certain issues involved—i.e., some of the questions raised therein—and place these conflicts into the terminology of contemporary medical ethics. For instance, a question of whether to treat a patient aggressively or to withhold treatment may be cast in terms of a conflict between the obligations or concepts of beneficence and nonmaleficence. This is meant simply to help the discussants to become comfortable with the common language and terminology of medical ethics. It is usually desirable that participants in discussions of clinical ethics become familiar with philosophical terminology but not fall in love with jargon. As ethicist Albert Jonsen put it, these terms are the "balloons" that provide a "wide view of the landscape and the horizons . . . far on all sides." They "escape the crowding details of human business" in favor of a distant clarity. Created by "imagination" and "loosely tethered to the ground," they gather weight as they take on the practical judgments of the front-line, clinical decision maker (Jonsen 1991). Our use of terms such as autonomy, beneficence, and nonmaleficence in conjunction with the rich detailed case and its description from various perspectives and outcomes, is intended to recognize the importance of moving beyond particulars as we struggle to define a moral solution. Of course, one of the lessons of case discussion is that these terms require a great deal of interpretation before they apply to the case at hand. Sometimes you will see that it has been helpful for us to coin terms such as "family autonomy" to help in situations where the more traditional "patient autonomy" is too narrow a concept to be helpful.

The sections of each case on the language and issues of the case, as well as the discussions that follow the cases, should certainly not be taken as exhaustive of the issues nor as providing definitive answers. Rather, they are meant to highlight some of the salient features and possible viewpoints on the case so as to provide a kind of "crib notes" for the discussion leader. We hope that these sections provide a starting point for the discussion and dialogue on these poignant and perplexing cases. But, the entire point of providing such thick description of each case is to provide room for identification of many issues and to facilitate reinterpretation. Similarly, we also provide many of the real-life outcomes of the cases so as to show what result certain actions may have. Nevertheless, one must resist the temptation to judge all the actions by the result. Sometimes, good actions have negative results and vice versa. We encourage discussion leaders to always pursue additional suggestions for action and to tap the moral imaginations of the participants for alternative outcomes. We simply wish to show that real life can often surprise us by the outcomes.

WHAT ABOUT ISSUES OF CONFIDENTIALITY?

This casebook is intended to help people run case discussions or other educational activities within their institutions. Because of this public distribution, we were especially concerned about the issue of confidentiality.

Confidentiality always poses a dilemma for educators in health-care ethics. On the one hand, we do not simply want to give in to the tendency that sees confidentiality as a defunct or "decrepit" concept (Siegler 1982). Despite the difficulties involved in preserving confidentiality, we cannot simply claim that all information gathered in a health-care institution is public property. Thus, some balance must be struck between preserving the richness available through "thick description" and purging the kind of details that would serve to expose the persons involved (Davis 1991).

To protect patient as well as provider confidentiality, the following steps have been taken:

1. The names of all those who have submitted cases appear in the Acknowledgments below. No names are listed with the cases. (Three of the cases were previously published with bylines in the CEP newsletter, *Community Ethics*. Because additional precautions were taken in these instances and the names have already been publicly linked, we note their original appearance in endnotes.)

2. The cases were altered to remove specific information that could be used to identify the institution from which they came. In some cases, this led to much greater changes than in others. In a few cases, this required virtually no alterations. However, facts such as gender were randomly varied from one case to the next.

3. Ultimately, time is the best protector of confidentiality. All of these cases were submitted at least two years prior to distribution, and most are fairly common scenarios. As such, more like them have probably taken place even within the very institutions from which they came.

REFERENCES

Dena S. Davis, 1991. "Rich cases: The ethics of thick description." *Hastings Center Report* 21(4): 12–17.

Albert R. Jonsen, 1991. "Of balloons and bicycles or the relationship between ethical theory and practical judgment." *Hastings Center Report* 21(5): 14–16.

Mark M. Siegler, 1982. "Confidentiality in medicine: A decrepit concept." *New England Journal of Medicine* 307:1518–21.

Acknowledgments and Participants

We wish to acknowledge the generous support of the Vira I. Heinz Endowment that was integral to this project. We also need to acknowledge Ms. Jody Chidester and Mr. Ryan Sauder for their help in the preparation of the manuscript. The exercise which gave rise to the book, a participant-driven educational exercise in continuing medical ethics, was initially suggested in 1992 by the CEP's former Consortium Ethicist Gretchen Aumann, RN, MSN, and Anne Medsgar, RN, MS, Evaluation Consultant. We thank them for suggesting the concept.

One of the cases included herein formed the basis of a journal article, and the collecting of cases was also the subject of a publication. We wish to thank the relevant editors and publishers for permission to reprint the cases and/or the discussion of the cases that appeared in the following articles:

Mark Kuczewski, Mark R. Wicclair, Robert M. Arnold, Rosa Lynn Pinkus, Gretchen M.E. Aumann, 1994. "Make my case: Ethics teaching and case presentations." *Journal of Clinical Ethics* 5(4): 310–15.

Mark G. Kuczewski, 1996. "Reconceiving the family: The process of consent in medical decision making." *Hastings Center Report* 26 (2): 30–37.

In alphabetical order follow the names of those who identified cases for this book. We wish to express our gratitude to each for sharing his or her experience.

Judith S. Black, M.D.
UPMC St. Margaret
Pittsburgh, PA

Darlette Cimino, R.N.
AUH Forbes Regional
Pittsburgh, PA

Elizabeth Chaitin, M.S.W., M.A.
UPMC Shadyside
Pittsburgh, PA

Michael DeVita, M.D.
University of Pittsburgh
Pittsburgh, PA

Patty Eppinger, C.M.S.C.
Jameson Memorial Hospital
New Castle, PA

Maryanne Fello, R.N., B.S.N.,
  M.Ed.
AUH Forbes Hospice
Pittsburgh, PA

Jeffrey Frye, M.D.
The Uniontown Hospital
Uniontown, PA

Marianne Garrity, R.N.
AUH Forbes Hospice
Pittsburgh, PA

Karen Gelston, M.S.W.
Bradford Hospital
Bradford, PA

Jeanne Graff, M.S.N.
United Community Hospital
Grove City, PA

Patricia Hillebrand, R.N.,
  C.N.S.
Indiana Hospital
Indiana, PA

Sandra Janaszek, R.N., M.S.N.
Meadeville Medical Center
Meadeville, PA

Mary Johnson, R.N.
Mercy Hospital
Pittsburgh, PA

Elayne Krahe, B.S.P.A.
Citizens General Hospital
New Kensington, PA

Mark Kuczewski, Ph.D.
Medical College of Wisconsin
Milwaukee, WI

Fran Kuhns, M.S.N.
Clarion Hospital
Clarion, PA

Leah Laffey, R.N., M.S.N.
UPMC St. Margaret
Pittsburgh, PA

Mary Jane Lesnick-Mertz, L.S.W.,
  A.C.S.W.
South Hills Health System
Pittsburgh, PA

John Lipson, M.D., M.B.A.
Indiana Hospital
Indiana, PA

Carol Lukoff, M.S.W.
Children's Hospital of Pittsburgh
Pittsburgh, PA

Patrick J. McCruden, M.T.S.
Marian Health Center
Sioux City, IA

Elizabeth Moore, M.S.W.
Sewickley Valley Hospital
Sewickley, PA

Cynthiane J. Morgenweck, M.D.
Medical College of Wisconsin
Milwaukee, WI

Alice Moskowitz
New York, NY

Teresa Nolan, M.D.
AUH Forbes Regional
Pittsburgh, PA

Joan Nypaver, B.S.N., C.R.R.N.
Hillside Rehabilitation Services
Warren, OH

Margaret Pavelek, R.N., B.S.N.
Jameson Memorial Hospital
New Castle, PA

William Prenatt, M.D.
United Community Hospital
Grove City, PA

Deborah Price, R.N., B.S.N.,
   M.H.A.
Bradford Hospital
Bradford, PA

Sarah Schlieper, L.S.W., C.C.M.
D.T. Watson Rehabilitation
   Services
Sewickley, PA

Jacqueline Sikina, R.N.
The Uniontown Hospital
Uniontown, PA

Tom Sobieralski, M.A.
Butler Memorial Hospital
Butler, PA

Sandy Thorpe, R.N.
The Uniontown Hospital
Uniontown, PA

Andrew Thurman, J.D., M.P.H.
Allegheny Health Education and
   Research Foundation
Pittsburgh, PA

Lillian Vendig-Bandyk, M.S.W.,
   M.P.H.
South Hills Health System
Pittsburgh, PA

Philip Williams, M.Div., S.T.M.
West Penn Hospital
Pittsburgh, PA

Mary Ellen Wyszomierski, M.D.
Latrobe Area Hospital
Latrobe, PA

Consent and Competence

Case One:
"He Doesn't Know What He's Saying"

KEY TERMS: *Competence to Give Informed Consent, Decision-Making Capacity, Advance Directives, Emergency Department Ethics*

NARRATIVE

Mr. J, a 65 year-old married man, presented at the emergency room in acute respiratory distress. He was anxious, alert, and gasping for air. His shortness of breath made talking with him difficult. He was accompanied by his wife and nephew.

Mr. J was fairly well known at this hospital, because he had been treated there for almost a decade for his chronic pulmonary disease. His illness progressed over the years to the point where he required assistance dressing and eating, and this assistance was provided by his wife who cared for him at home. Mr. J had been admitted to the hospital 10 months before, at which time he was intubated and placed on a respirator. Later there was great difficulty weaning the patient from the machine, but the pulmonologist managed to do so after two weeks. According to the family, Mr. J expressed strong feelings at that time that he should never be placed on a ventilator again.

During the current admission, Mrs. J and her nephew spoke with the attending physician in the emergency department while Mr. J was taken to the treatment room. They explained what they believed to be the wishes of the patient. That is, they asked that Mr. J be given any helpful medications but not intubated. They also asked that his code status be Do-Not-Resuscitate (DNR). The family said that Mr. J should be made "comfortable" and that necessary medications could be given to him.

The family did not enter the treatment room with the physician. The physician examined the patient, and in the presence of nursing staff and respiratory therapists, the physician explained to Mr. J the need for intubation. Mr. J agreed to this by nodding his head "yes." This process took place quickly due to the emergency conditions. Mr. J was intubated and placed on a ventilator within 10 minutes of admission. Upon learning of the intubation, the family became very upset.

THE LANGUAGE AND ISSUES OF THE CASE

Several problems raise their heads. Clearly this case will be discussed in terms of the patient's right to make his own decision, i.e., patient autonomy. But whether this is an autonomous decision will require placing several matters in context, namely:

1. determining the patient's capacity to consent to treatment ("competence");
2. identifying the role of previous directions ("advance directives") in treatment decisions;
3. deciding the role of family or surrogates in interpreting the wishes of a patient.

PERSPECTIVES AND KEY POINTS OF VIEW

ER Physician: The physician was reluctant to take the family's initial request at face value. He believed that a patient who presents at the ER should receive the kind of care that is standard in such emergency situations. Thus, he has the normal presumption to treat in the emergency situation. Furthermore, he was also reluctant to take the family's request at face value since the patient was conscious. Although competence is at issue, the physician believed that he should presume the patient to be competent to consent to life-saving interventions unless clearly shown otherwise. After the fact, the physician wondered whether he had done the right thing.

The Family (Mrs. J and Nephew): The family members believed that they knew the patient's real wishes because they had a long period over which to discuss the future course of treatment. They also believe that if Mr. J contradicted what they believed to be his genuine wishes, it must be due to hypoxia or the coercive atmosphere of the treatment room. They dreaded the possibility that the prolonged agony of the previous difficult weaning period would be repeated. Mr. J was generally conscious through those attempts, and they watched the patient linger in fear and suffering for two weeks. They also feared that they would be "killing" Mr. J if they withdrew the respirator after unsuccessful weaning attempts, but that it would have been acceptable if Mr. J had not been started on the mechanical ventilation in the first place. They believe that the ER physician had betrayed them and undermined their familial role as the interpreters of the patient's wishes.

POSSIBLE ALTERNATIVE ENDINGS

The main alternative course of action open at the time of admission would have had one or both members of the family accompanying the patient into the treatment room for the "informed consent" conversation. If the disorientation that the medical environment induces and the patient's fear of abandonment are real factors, having familial support in that environment might provide more insight into the patient's true wishes. However, one must be careful not to allow the family to make the competency determination on the basis of whether the patient says what they would like to hear.

Furthermore, the best alternatives might have been preventive ones that took place before this dilemma occurred. For instance, after the last discharge from the hospital, the patient and family, in concert with the patient's attending physician, could have developed documentation and a more comprehensive plan for dealing with this type of crisis. This plan might well have included some option other than admission via the emergency room.

COMMENTARY

This case is of a kind that is increasingly replicated in emergency rooms around the country. The *Hastings Center Report* (Silverman, et al. 1992) describes a similar situation involving the use of a living will. However, whether a living will document is involved or the advance directive is verbal does not change the issues involved. These cases pit prior directions by the patient against a present situation in which it is not clear if those directions apply.

In this case, the patient's current capacity to consent to treatment is at issue. If he is able to consent, then his prior directions do not matter. Prior directives do not surpass the patient's right to give contemporaneous consent.

Some consensus exists on this kind of case, and, in this case, that consensus supports the actions of the ER physician and health-care team (Iserson 1996). Adult patients are presumed to be competent until shown to be otherwise (Meisel, Grenvik, et al. 1986; Buchanan and Brock 1989, 21). Furthermore, when in serious doubt, it is obviously appropriate to err on the side of life (President's Commission 1983, 3). This principle is reflected in the advance directive statutes of many states. For instance, even if the patient was deemed incompetent, the Pennsylvania Advance Directive for Health Care Act counsels the physician to accept the patient's override of the prior directive if the patient wishes to revoke it (Meisel and Dorst 1992a). So, the ethical and legal consensus is on the side of allowing this patient to consent to treatment. Not to do so is to make advance directives into contractual death warrants. The legal and ethical consensus on this point is really no more than an extension of the risk-related standard of patient competence to consent to treatment (President's Commission 1982, 60–62; Drane 1984, 1985).

Allowing the family to accompany the patient into the treatment room could be helpful in determining the correct treatment decision and also in keeping the patient calm and less fearful throughout the treatment process. It is likely that it would also have prevented the family coming to feel that they had been betrayed. Nevertheless, if a conflict did result between the patient and family in the treatment room, good sense would counsel honoring the wishes of the patient.

Clearly, the only truly satisfactory solution to this type of issue is good advance planning and consultation prior to the emergent event (Forrow, Arnold, and Parker 1993). Documentation of the patient's wishes over time and development of a plan to deal with the onset of crisis that provides clear instructions for the health-care workers are essential. Discussing with the patient that he or she may be excited or upset at the time of the emergency and identifying ways to overcome the element of fear can be invaluable. There is no substitute for talking to the patient at the time of treatment, but such documentation will help to frame the conversation and provide context for the decisions. However, even with good advance planning, we must be aware that situations such as this one will present themselves and will contain an implicit conflict between a presumption in favor of treatment and a desire to serve the patient's long-term goals. This may simply be one of the special problems that arise by the very nature of emergency medicine (Derse 1990, Iserson 1996).

Finally, despite the psychological difficulties in withdrawing life-sustaining treatment, there is no established moral or legal distinction between withholding and withdrawing treatment. In this case, the physician did well to start the treatment because such treatment could be withdrawn later after a more thorough investigation was made into the wishes of the patient.

REFERENCES

Allen E. Buchanan, Dan W. Brock, 1989. *Deciding for others: The ethics of surrogate decision making.* New York: Cambridge University Press.

Arthur R. Derse, 1990. "Ethics emergent." *Annals of Emergency Medicine* 19(2): 210–12.

James F. Drane, 1984. "Competency to give informed consent." *Journal of the American Medical Association* 252(7):925–27.

James F. Drane, 1985. "The many faces of competency." *Hastings Center Report* 15(2):17–21.

Lachlan Forrow, Robert M. Arnold, Lisa S. Parker, 1993. "Preventive ethics: Expanding the horizon of clinical ethics." *Journal of Clinical Ethics* 4(4):287–94.

Kenneth V. Iserson, 1996. "Withholding and withdrawing medical treatment: An emergency medicine perspective." *Annals of Emergency Medicine* 28(1): 51–54.

Alan Meisel, Ake Grenvik, Rosa Lynn Pinkus, James V. Snyder, 1986. "Hospital guidelines for deciding about life-sustaining treatment: Dealing with health "Limbo." *Critical Care Medicine* 14(3):239–46.

Alan Meisel, Stanley K. Dorst, 1992a. "Living wills given life in Pa." *Pennsylvania Law Journal* 15(29):5, 29.

President's Commission for the Study of Ethical Problems in Medicine and Biomedical and Behavioral Research, 1982. *Making health care decisions*, Vol. 1, Washington, DC: U.S. Government Printing Office.

President's Commission for the Study of Ethical Problems in Medicine and Biomedical and Behavioral Research, 1983. *Deciding to forego life-sustaining treatment*. Washington, DC: U.S. Government Printing Office.

Lewis M. Silverman, Manette Dennis, Fenella Rouse, David A. Smith, 1992. Commentaries on "Whether no means no." *Hastings Center Report* 22(2): 26–27.

Case Two:
Consent and the Elderly

KEY TERMS: *Competence, Informed Consent, Ageism, Power of Attorney, Durable Power of Attorney for Health Care (DPAHC)*

NARRATIVE

Mrs. F is an 84 year-old resident of a local nursing facility who was evaluated in the emergency room after sustaining a fall in the bathroom. She has had multiple medical problems in the past, none of which have been particularly debilitating. She has a history of hypertension, depression, arthritis, hyperthyroidism, and a vague diagnosis of senile dementia.

Upon falling in the bathroom, Mrs. F apparently struck her head and sustained a large hematoma and a laceration. She was evaluated by the staff of the nursing facility and found to be alert and oriented. Because of the laceration, she was transferred to the emergency room for evaluation. In the emergency room, a routine CT scan of the head was obtained and revealed a rather large subdural hematoma compressing the ventricles and pushing on the brain. In spite of this finding, Mrs. F seemed to be her usual self and was aware that she was in the emergency room and was conversing easily with the staff there. It was explained to her that she had a condition that could not be treated at the community hospital and that she required transfer to a tertiary care facility. She accepted this and told the emergency room physician that it would be okay to transfer her.

On arrival at the emergency room of the tertiary care facility, Mrs. F was evaluated by a neurosurgeon. At that time, the patient was complaining of a headache. She related that she knew she was at a different hospital and was not in the nursing home. She was unable to give any details as to what had happened to her but was able to relay that she had fallen and struck her head. Neurological examination revealed she had decreased motor strength of the right side and somewhat garbled speech. The neurosurgeon needed to determine whether Mrs. F should undergo a burr hole to drain her subdural hematoma to relieve the pressure from the brain or return her to the nursing home and monitor her in the hope that the clot would resolve.

While staying at the nursing home, Mrs. F was noted by the staff to be an alert and gregarious elderly woman who "got around" well. She performed most of her activities of daily living with minimal assistance. She was oriented at all times. While at the nursing home, Mrs. F had completed an advance directive. This advance directive stated that "if she were ever terminally ill or permanently unconscious, life-prolonging measures such as cardiac resuscitation, ventilatory support, and artificial nutrition and hydration should be withheld." The patient also requested comfort measures if she should become debilitated. Mrs. F designated her nephew as her power of attorney. The power of attorney was solely for financial transactions and did not impart health-care decision-making powers to the nephew. Discovered after the fact was that Mrs. F had a sister. Unfortunately, the staff at the nursing home facility were unaware of this sister's existence. Her husband was deceased and she had no children.

At this point, the neurosurgeon elected to contact Mrs. F's power of attorney, her nephew. He believed this was her only living relative. The neurosurgeon discussed Mrs. F's case with her nephew at some length and relayed to him that Mrs. F had an advance directive. He explained the critical nature of Mrs. F's condition and the potentially devastating outcome should surgery not be performed.

Mrs. F's nephew was unsure as to how to proceed at that time. It is not clear if he understood the gravity of the situation or the fact that a burr hole would relieve the pressure on Mrs. F's brain. At this point, a decision was made to return the patient to the nursing home on anticonvulsant medications and to perform no surgical intervention.

THE LANGUAGE AND ISSUES OF THE CASE

This case raises a variety of issues, depending on which point in Mrs. F's treatment one focuses and on whom one focuses, e.g., the neurosurgeon, the patient's attending physician, the nursing home staff. Questions of informed consent loom large early, and then questions regarding decision-making capacity and the naming of an appropriate surrogate take precedence later. We can ask:

1. Is a surrogate decision maker necessary in this case or was Mrs. F's autonomy violated by not being included in a discussion of her medical condition and potential treatments?
2. If a surrogate decision maker was necessary, was the appropriate surrogate Mrs. F's nephew who was her power of attorney for financial matters?
3. Did the neurosurgeon in this case make a prejudiced determination of Mrs. F's quality of life prior to her fall and thereby

base decisions upon faulty assumptions about her? Or was he practicing the standard of care for the treatment of a hematoma in a patient of her age?

4. Were there others in this patient's life, e.g., nursing home staff, her primary care physician, who should have played a larger role in the decision-making process?

PERSPECTIVES AND KEY POINTS OF VIEW

The Patient: We have no idea what she actually thought. She was not really asked.

The Nursing Home Staff: The staff who knew Mrs. F at the nursing home described her as capable of making her own decisions because she was always quite conversant and self-directing. They were outraged that the patient did not undergo surgery and that they were left out of the decision-making process. They also now have an added burden to monitor her closely while the clot is resolving.

The Nephew: He was the financial power of attorney and was not comfortable with being asked to make health-care decisions concerning his aunt. It was his feeling that the health-care decisions should be left up to the physicians involved and that they would know best what to do with his aunt.

The Neurosurgeon: He believed the patient was incompetent to make treatment decisions. This neurosurgeon felt burdened because he had to lead the patient's surrogate in making a decision to operate or not. The nephew did not have a clear preference and so, the neurosurgeon believed he must provide the decision. He did not think she was a good candidate for surgery and also knew that, given time, the clot could resolve without further harm to the patient.

POSSIBLE ALTERNATIVE ENDINGS

A competent patient always has a right to be included in the process of treatment decision making. The neurosurgeon did not include the patient in the discussion concerning her condition and potential outcomes. Of course, when talking with an injured patient, decision-making capacity can be difficult to assess and the patient's life story, the narrative background against which treatment choices must make sense, is sometimes hidden. Family can often provide crucial insights, but this patient's nephew does not seem equipped to be of much aid nor does he desire to play a decisive role. The best way to resolve this case probably would have been for the neurosurgeon to contact either the nursing home facility or the patient's primary care attending physician. Had he, at the point of indecision, contacted the facility or the patient's primary care physician, he would have obtained a better understanding of the patient's previous standard of health and, therefore, what functional status she might again achieve through aggressive treatment. He would have been able to rely on those people who best know the patient in making a decision as to whether to proceed with surgery.

WHAT ACTUALLY HAPPENED

Mrs. F was returned to the nursing home facility. One day later, she was evaluated by her primary care physician. At that time, she was semi-comatose. She was totally paralyzed on her right side and had a ragged breathing pattern. The attending physician contacted Mrs. F's nephew to discuss her condition. Mrs. F's nephew, at this point, said that he wanted her to undergo the surgery if the attending physician felt that any of the symptoms were reversible. Given her grave respiratory and neurological status, the attending physician felt that it would be inappropriate to pursue surgery. Mrs. F was therefore maintained on anticonvulsant medications and observed. In two weeks time, Mrs. F was again able to swallow and was opening her eyes and responding to simple commands. Since there was some improvement in her condition and in subsequent CT scans, a second neurosurgical consultation was obtained. This consultant's opinion was that Mrs. F's subdural hematoma was resolving and she would not require surgery. After one month, Mrs. F was able to sit unassisted, was again using her right side, and was able to walk a few steps. Although not quite the same, she became alert and oriented to her surroundings and able to carry on conversations with the nursing facility staff.

COMMENTARY

This case is a vivid reminder that a patient has the right to be in control of his or her health-care decisions. That is, the patient must give informed consent before any major procedure can be performed and the patient should be a party to the entire decision-making process. If the patient's capacity to participate is impaired, then the substituted judgment standard of decision making should be employed. This means that a person who knows the patient's wishes and values well must try to choose for the patient as the patient would. In real life, the two standards often work together when we are not sure about level of impairment of the patient's decision-making capacity. When we do not employ this framework for decision making, the door is open to medical paternalism. Then, decisions that reflect the biases, preferences, and oftentimes, the good professional judgment of the caregivers may govern the outcome (Pinkus 1996). In this case, a caregiver who did not know the patient prior to admission proceeded to withhold aggressive treatment on the basis of his own determination of the patient's "best interest" (President's Commission 1982). As we have seen, he was probably mistaken in his judgment as to what the patient would have wanted although the results were not tragic.

In this case, both the informed consent approach to medical decision making and the substituted judgment standard should have worked together. It is not clear if the patient lacked the capacity to make a decision regarding a procedure to remove the subdural hematoma. It is clear, however, that the surrogate chosen by the neurosurgeon did not know what the patient would have wanted. Had the physician been more savvy in his application of the substituted judgment standard, he would probably have realized that Mrs. F's nephew was not the best surrogate since he did not feel comfortable speaking in her stead. Perhaps the patient's regular attending physician or the nursing home staff should have been involved in the decision-making process (Kuczewski 1999). As we have seen, the staff at the nursing facility, in fact, had an idea of what the patient would have wanted.

Moreover, if application of the substituted judgment standard is not viable due to difficulty in ascertaining the appropriate surrogate, then best interests of the patient should be considered. The draining of a subdural hematoma is a relatively benign procedure with a potentially tremendous benefit. It would seem in this case that the patient's best interest would have been to undergo the procedure. We can surmise that the neurosurgeon mistakenly thought Mrs. F to be more frail and sickly than was actually her baseline state. He probably also assumed that her living will was further evidence that her life was burdensome to her and death would be welcome. As a result, he misidentified her interests.

In sum, providers must be careful not to read their biases, ageist or otherwise, into particular cases (Greene, et al. 1986; Wicclair 1993, 80–120). This is one reason why patients have a right to participate in their care. Patients are probably better at safeguarding their own interests than are their caregivers, however well intentioned. The patient has the right to define her needs and to guide her health-care decisions unless it is shown that she is incapacitated in this regard. Then, it is the responsibility of the health-care professional to educate the patient's surrogate and to make every possible effort to ascertain the patient's wishes concerning his or her health care.

REFERENCES

Michele G. Greene, Ronald Adelman, Rita Charon, Susie Hoffman, 1986. "Ageism in the medical encounter: An exploratory study of the doctor–elderly patient relationship." *Language and Communication* 6(½):113–24.

Mark G. Kuczewski, 1999. "Ethics in long-term care: Are the principles different?" *Theoretical Medicine and Bioethics* 20(1).

Rosa Lynn B. Pinkus, 1996. "Politics, paternalism, and the rise of the neurosurgeon: The evolution of moral reasoning." *Medical Humanities Review* 10(2): 20–44.

President's Commission for the Study of Ethical Problems in Medicine and Biomedical and Behavioral Research, 1982. *Making health care decisions*, Vol. 1, Washington, DC: U.S. Government Printing Office.

Mark R. Wicclair, 1993. *Ethics and the elderly.* New York: Oxford University Press.

Case Three:
Caring for the Indecisive Patient: No Longer Secret but Still a Problem

KEY TERMS: *Autonomy, Surrogate Decision Making, Ethics Committees, Pain Management*

NARRATIVE

Mrs. K is a 64 year-old woman who was admitted to the hospital with a nine-day history of a painful and discolored left middle toe. At the time of admission she also reported a 50-pound weight loss, nausea, decreased appetite and vomiting. Her past medical history was significant for a spinal fusion about 18 months before. Since that time, the patient had had chronic pain and been functionally dependent on her husband for daily care. Mr. K was her only immediate family member. The patient's family history showed that both her father and paternal grandfather died of pancreatic cancer. One had a "quiet death," the other did not.

Evaluation of Mrs. K's weight loss revealed metastatic adenocarcinoma of the pancreas. She initially underwent a CT scan of the abdomen that showed metastatic lesions to the liver and a mass in the pancreas. These findings were confirmed by a CT-guided biopsy. The consulting oncologist noted in the chart that the patient said her main concern was "quality" in her final days of life. He indicated the most pressing issue to decide was whether or not to proceed with amputation of the leg. The oncologist did not want to consider any further therapeutic intervention to treat the cancer until after this surgical procedure which was necessitated by her ischemic foot.

During the hospitalization the limited necrotic area of the left foot progressed to involve the entire left foot and resulted in increased pain. Mrs. K was asked to consider an amputation of her left leg above the knee. The physician brought up this issue on the same day that the oncologist informed her of her diagnosis of pancreatic cancer. At that point in time, she could not make any decisions, and it wasn't until five days later that she agreed to the amputation.

Mrs. K's hospital course was complicated by pneumonia, hyponatremia of unknown etiology, malnutrition, intermittent delirium, hypothyroidism, and congestive heart failure. She was refusing blood work, declining to eat, and would not take her medications for her hypothy-roidism and congestive heart failure. She also pulled her central line.

During her hospitalization she indicated several times that she wished to "die quietly." Mrs. K also had an advance directive. On this directive, she indicated that when she was permanently unconscious or terminally ill, cardiopulmonary resuscitation, respirators, dialysis, feeding tube, radiation, or chemotherapy should be withheld or with-drawn. When asked about decisions such as treating pneumonia, IV hydration, and antibiotics, she stated, "I can't decide. My mind is blank." After talking with her attending physician, Mrs. K often agreed to treatments she had previously refused.

The code status form was completed for "comfort measures only." Social Service was consulted to assist in discharge planning to a long-term-care facility. The transfer to the long-term-care facility was compli-cated by the fact Mrs. K had pneumonia for which she was intermittently refusing treatment.

THE LANGUAGE AND ISSUES OF THE CASE

As in most cases of treatment decision making with a conscious patient, this case is likely to be discussed in terms of respecting the autonomy of the patient and her right of self-determination. Of course, when it is unclear just what the patient would want, the issue of the patient's decision-making capacity or competence comes to the fore. But any savvy reader will know that the problems in this case will not resolve simply by making a determination of that capacity. More specific causes for her vacillation need to be identified, and a process of sup-porting this patient through the decision-making process must evolve. Some specific questions might be useful in shaping this process:

1. Is Mrs. K's indecisiveness fear-related? That is, is it general fear of death or related to what she had experienced with her father and grandfather dying of pancreatic cancer?
2. Why does Mrs. K often agree to treatment after discussions with her attending physician? Does he elicit what she really wants to do? Does she agree just to please her doctor? Or is Mrs. K being pressured to change her decisions?
3. If no clear cause for her vacillation can be identified, does that mean Mrs. K is not competent to make her own decisions re-garding care? That is, does her indecisiveness equal a lack of ca-pacity? If so, is Mr. K the legitimate surrogate decision maker? If he is also indecisive, does that mean he is incompetent to serve as the surrogate?

4. Does the attending physician have the knowledge base and experience to prescribe optimal pain management control for this terminally ill patient?
5. Has hospice care, which the husband has mentioned, been thoroughly investigated for an established diagnosis of metastatic pancreatic cancer?

PERSPECTIVES AND KEY POINTS OF VIEW

Nursing Staff: The nursing staff was concerned that the patient's pain was not being adequately controlled. Furthermore they believed that this was a symptom of a larger problem, i.e., no clear treatment goals had been developed. They understood that this was partially due to the vacillation of the patient and wished to get the patient's assistance in making a decision. However, they were wary of involving Mr. K in this process, because they had smelled alcohol on his breath and were suspicious that he might not have the patient's best interest at heart.

Attending Physician: The attending physician had indicated the patient was terminal but also had particular reversible conditions. As the attending physician, he felt obligated legally to treat reversible conditions unless the patient steadfastly refused such treatment. He was concerned that reimbursement for hospital days would be denied if no treatment was given and that he would be delivering suboptimal care if he discharged the patient to the extended care facility with active treatable conditions. Although he sometimes got the patient to agree to start a course of treatment for certain ailments, he had been unable to elicit long-lasting decisions from the patient or the husband. In the area of pain control, he felt there was significant risk that increased narcotics for pain would "do her in."

The Social Worker: The social worker had raised a concern that the husband smelled of alcohol while visiting. Placement for the patient in an extended care facility was available but was awaiting medical clearance. The social worker was unclear what the patient's prognosis was and unsure if the patient's prognosis qualified her for hospice care. The social worker had difficulty dealing with Mr. and Mrs. K because of their indecisiveness. The social worker also observed the patient occasionally had paranoid thoughts about the hospital staff.

Mr. K: The husband is the only immediate family, and he wished for his wife to receive comfort measures only. He understood that it would be necessary to maintain need for skilled nursing if nursing home financial coverage was to remain in effect.

POSSIBLE ALTERNATIVE ENDINGS

One month after hospitalization an ethics consultation was requested by the nursing staff. A consultant met with the nurse who requested the consult and also spoke individually with the attending physician, the husband, and patient. The ethics team suggested the following:

1. Hold a team meeting with the attending physician, primary nurse, patient, husband, and social worker to define goals so all are aware of all perspectives involved. Given the patient's and husband's difficulty with decisions, concrete, specific issues should be addressed: (a) Do you want pneumonia treated? In order to treat pneumonia adequately, what would be required, what would be expected if not treated, and alternatives to provide comfort (e.g., respiratory distress—subcutaneous morphine, oxygen, etc.); (b) possible pain management alternatives including risks (e.g., continue current plan with increased frequency, morphine drip—central IV line would probably be necessary, topical Fentanlyl, combination of above, etc.)
2. Assure that clearly written or dictated summary of issues is sent to those providing care after hospital discharge.

WHAT ACTUALLY HAPPENED

Mrs. K continued to refuse blood work and the placement of a central line for IV hydration. The attending physician increased the frequency and amount of pain medication. The recommendations of the ethics committee were then partially followed. That is, there was a family conference attended by the nurse who requested the consultation, the hospital social worker, and the patient and her husband. The attending physician did not participate. After this meeting, Mr. and Mrs. K decided on a long-term-care facility, and the patient was transferred five days after the ethics consult to that facility for supportive care. The patient died ten days after the transfer.

COMMENTARY

This case illustrates many of the classic issues in clinical medical ethics. The caregivers wish to respect the patient's autonomy. However, doing so is not simple. The patient's wishes are changeable due to disorientation caused by the illness, the need to process her situation, cognitively and emotionally, and so forth. It is not immediately obvious how the physician should influence the process. On the one hand, he has a duty to help the patient, i.e., beneficence. The attending physician in this case interprets that duty in terms of treating reversible conditions. The nursing staff suspects that this view is inconsistent with coherent treatment goals that "treat the whole patient" by also taking into account the duty not to harm the patient (nonmaleficence). It is important that the physician and the nursing staff have an opportunity to see each other's perspectives. And it is possible that underlying this difference of viewpoints is a fear by the physician that "allowing" to die is "causing" death, and this question should be addressed directly by an ethics consultant familiar with these distinctions (Clouser 1977; President's Commission 1983, 60–90; Kuczewski 1998).

Of course, if the patient clearly knew what she wanted, the physician would probably honor it. One can sympathize with the patient's vacillation. She has a variety of ailments that make her very sick, they are being diagnosed within hours or days of each other, and some of them, such as her cancer, have a variety of affective implications. Just as the patient is ready to make one momentous decision (amputation), news of another, even more serious illness (adenocarcinoma) is presented.

The ethics committee's strategy makes sense. The patient and her husband should process this information for a while but, at some point, there needs to be a conference at which the options are clarified and goals selected. Setting such a decision point often helps the patient to make decisions. Such conferences present an opportunity to be sure that the health-care team is not working at cross purposes and that all have access to the same information. Additionally, at such a conference different members of the health-care team may provide reassurance to the patient that forgoing treatment will not lead to her abandonment by the caregivers. This message may not be coming through in the physician-patient discussions.

It is also important that we not overstate the degree of vacillation this patient was exhibiting. The narrative of the case suggests that the patient consistently valued a "quiet death" and was mainly concerned about her "quality of life." The difficulty in this case probably stems from translating those general values or treatment goals into answers to the specific questions concerning particular treatments. Patients are not experts concerning medical treatments; health-care professionals are. However, patients know their own values or goals best, although elaborating what such things as a "quiet death" mean can be helped along considerably by dialogue between the patient and the health-care professionals.

Unfortunately, the recommendations of the ethics consultants focused on both the goals and the particular treatment decisions. The goals need to be paramount. Those must be explored first in a nondirective way in order to understand what the patient wants and wishes to avoid. Then, the health-care professionals can be more directive in recommending the treatment plan that will best bring about these goals. In other words, too much emphasis was being put on "what" the patient wanted and not nearly enough on "why" she might want it (Forrow 1994).

This case also raised the issue of whether or not all medical physicians are up-to-date with treating cancer pain and providing optimal pain management (Meier, et al. 1997; Sachs, et al. 1995; Hill 1993; Portenoy 1993; Weissman 1996). This sensitive issue was raised by the ethics committee. If the ethics committee is to recommend a pain management consultation or to develop a subcommittee to review pain management, is this in effect telling the physicians how to practice? Will this, in turn, deter physicians from utilizing the ethics committee for consultations?

In sum, the difficulty in this case is twofold. (a) There is the murky "stuff of ethics" properly speaking. This material includes coming to understand the patient's values, facilitating translation of values into treatment goals, and then developing a specific treatment plan that serves those ends. (b) Then, there is simply the practical matter of being sure that the patient receives the appropriate kind and quality of care whether that be aggressive in nature, strictly palliative, or something in between. Although these two difficulties seem clear enough, and they are easily analyzed by medical and medical ethics texts, as this case points out, in practice they may always be "still a problem" (Youngner 1987).

REFERENCES

K. Danner Clouser, 1977. "Allowing or causing: Another look." *Annals of Internal Medicine* 87(5):622–624.

Lachlan Forrow, 1994. "The green eggs and ham phenomenon." *Hastings Center Report* 24(6):S29–S32.

C. Stratton Hill, Jr., 1993. "The barriers to adequate pain management with opioid analgesics." *Seminars in Oncology* 20(2):S1,1–5.

Mark G. Kuczewski, 1998. "Physician-assisted death: Can philosophical bioethics aid social policy?" *Cambridge Quarterly of Healthcare Ethics* 7(4): 339–47.

Diane E. Meier, Sean R. Morrison, Christine K. Cassel, 1997. "Improving palliative care." *Annals of Internal Medicine* 127(3):225–30.

Russell K. Portenoy, 1993. "Cancer pain management." *Seminars in Oncology* 20(2):S1,19–35.

President's Commission for the Study of Ethical Problems in Medicine and Biomedical and Behavioral Research, 1983. *Deciding to forego life-sustaining treatment*. Washington, DC: U.S. Government Printing Office.

Greg A. Sachs, Judith C. Ahronheim, Jill A. Rhymes, Ladislav Volicer, Joanne Lynn, 1995. "Good care of dying patients: The alternative to physician-assisted suicide and euthanasia." *Journal of the American Geriatrics Society* 43:553–62.

David E. Weissman, 1996. "Cancer pain education for physicians in practice: Establishing a new paradigm." *Journal of Pain and Symptom Management* 12(6):364–71.

Stuart J. Youngner, 1987. "Do-not-resuscitate orders: No longer secret, but still a problem." *Hastings Center Report* 17(1):24–33.

FOR FURTHER READING

Joy Kroeger-Mappes, 1996. "Ethical dilemmas for nurses: Physician's orders versus patient's rights." In Thomas A. Mappes, David DeGrazia, eds. *Biomedical Ethics*, 4th ed., pp. 139–46.

Robert Veatch, 1987. "The dying cancer patient." *Case Studies in Medical Ethics*. Philadelphia PA: Lippincott, pp. 44–48.

James L. Bernat, Bernard Gert, R. Peter Mogielnicky, "Patient refusal of hydration and nutrition: An alternative to physician-assisted suicide or voluntary active euthanasia." *Archives of Internal Medicine* 153:2723–28, 1993.

Case Four:
Withdrawing Treatment: Easier Said Than Done

KEY TERMS: *Decision-Making Capacity, Forgoing Treatment, Suicide, Ethics Committees, Ethics Consultation*

NARRATIVE

The patient, Mrs. M, was a 54 year-old woman who was transferred to this tertiary care hospital's Critical Care Unit (CCU) from an outlying community hospital with a principle diagnosis of acute anterior wall myocardial infarction (MI), i.e., a heart attack. Secondary diagnoses were acute pancreatitis, disseminated intravascular coagulation, acute respiratory failure, acute renal failure, and lactic acidosis. The patient was placed on a ventilator. Due to medication and her increasing medical problems, she was only periodically alert, but responsive when directly addressed. There were no written advance directives.

Mrs. M was hospitalized in 1990 for acute pancreatitis. She also had a psychiatric history of anxiety and depression and had been consistently treated with Haldol and Prozac for several years. Mrs. M attempted suicide about ten years ago.

Her family consisted of a supportive husband (Mr. M), an adult daughter (Martha), the daughter's husband, and a 15-year-old granddaughter (Rachel). The M's have a son (Jake) who lived in the Midwest. He wasn't present at the hospital. Jake also had a history of depression and suicide attempts. The family informed him of his mother's serious condition but purposely kept him out of the decision-making loop, fearing his acting out if he saw his mother fulfilling his possible latent wish. Mr. M and Martha consistently voiced agreement that Mrs. M should make her own decision regarding treatment or a terminal wean. Mr. M said that his wife and he had talked about potential end-of-life situations. She was clear that she did not want to be kept alive if it meant living in a more debilitated state or if the quality of her life would be compromised more than it already had been.

The first three days of hospitalization the patient was consistently aware and responsive. She was presented with the possibility of pancreatic surgery to relieve her excruciating pancreatitis or with drug treatments. She was told that surgery had a high risk of mortality with less than 50 percent chance she would come out of the OR alive. Recovery would require extensive respiratory care with possible placement for a period of time in an extended care facility where she would be in a program for redevelopment of ADL skills (Activities of Daily Living). Within these first three days it also became clear that she would have to have dialysis. Mrs. M declined more medical intervention and expressed a desire to discontinue ventilator support.

With Mrs. M's decision and the support of her husband and daughter, the attending physician agreed to a terminal wean. In a further phone conversation with the daughter on the day prior to the scheduled wean (the fourth day of hospitalization), the attending physician hesitated on the matter and called an ethics consult. The physician was concerned about Mrs. M's age and her potential to rally medically. The attending physician thought that treatment should clearly be "futile" before it was stopped, and he was not sure that this was presently the case. He was also concerned about Mrs. M's past history and her ongoing treatment for depression. He wondered whether her decision might be a kind of physician-assisted suicide. He also began to question the patient's decision-making capacity, i.e., competence.

At this point, Mr. M and Martha became angry and distraught about the seeming reversal and the calling of "more people," i.e., the ethics committee. The husband and daughter had already communicated to Mrs. M that her decision was to be honored. They were also initiating their own anticipatory grief process prior to this apparent delay and potential reversal. The ambivalence in decision making moved this process into conflict and indecisiveness.

THE LANGUAGE AND ISSUES OF THE CASE

Once again, we have questions regarding the decision-making capacity of a conscious patient. But this time any real questions about her competence will be based on an alleged psychiatric disorder rather than cognitive deficits. To some degree, we see a struggle taking place about the label to be applied to this decision of the patient, i.e., is it better labeled "suicide" or "forgoing treatment"? It is this struggle that seems to be raising questions in the mind of the physician concerning whether it will be a violation of his professional integrity to comply with the patient's wishes. As we have heard from his conversation with the patient's daughter, he believes that the appropriate label for this action is a function not only of the patient's intent but also the relative "futility" of the treatment being declined. Some specific questions this physician may need answer to include:

1. Should the patient's wishes and decisions be taken at face value without psychiatric evaluation? Should the severity of her medical condition automatically cast doubt on her decision-making capacity?
2. Should the physician abide by the wishes of the patient even if he has medical and ethical concerns or should he have transferred care to another physician who had fewer problems with the situation?
3. What does "futility" mean in a case like this?
4. Whose decision is this? Does family support for a position such as this one add to its moral acceptability?
5. Can an ethics consultation that is called by the attending physician be refused by the patient and family?

PERSPECTIVES AND KEY POINTS OF VIEW

Mrs. M: Throughout her hospitalization, she had consistently communicated that she wanted no treatment to prolong her life. She wanted to be weaned off the ventilator. Living a sedentary life with increasing limitations on what she might be able to do or enjoy did not appeal to Mrs. M. She was a voracious reader and limitations on such sedate activities were more than she could bear. Her family described her as no longer in love with life as such, but as "tolerating" it.

Mr. M (husband): He loved his wife and even though he did not want to lose her, he maintained that her right to make her own decision was primary. He recounted their conversations about end-of-her-life decisions in which Mrs. M was clearly opposed to unnecessary prolongation of her life, even with a small medical possibility of recovery. Mr. M maintained two principal values to which the whole family steadfastly ascribed: promise keeping and not lying. He made a promise to abide by her wishes. He did not want to see himself or be seen as lying. Mr. M feared that the delay, caused by the physician, threatened to make it appear to Mrs. M that he was withholding the truth from her and not carrying out her wishes. Promising to abide by his wife's wishes and decisions had a higher value than maintaining her life even with a low potential recovery.

Martha (daughter): She loved her mother and even though there were some unresolved mother/daughter issues, she held to the values her father and mother espoused. She was adamant in supporting her mother's decision and resented the questioning of her mother's competency. She wanted to honor her mother and get on with the anticipatory grief process, to be with her mother in her dying. She, like her father, was hostile toward the physician and ethics committee for delaying and potentially reversing what appeared to be an agreed upon decision.

Attending Physician: He had second thoughts. He knew the potential for long-term survival was low. Although the multiple consultations were in conflict about which organs might recover, the overall medical picture was bleak. Nevertheless, he was concerned that this was not futile care and feared that limiting treatment might be physician-assisted suicide. He raised competency issues and then became more ethically unsure of the decision.

Nursing Staff: Nursing was continuing to provide good care. The patient's nurses clearly supported the patient and family. They were becoming irritated with the physician's and consultants' "part versus whole" approach to medical care and the delay in carrying out the patient's decision.

WHAT ACTUALLY HAPPENED

The chaplain had been in conversation with the family, the patient, and the attending physician. On the fourth day of hospitalization, there appeared to be agreement among all to meet the following morning to exchange views and review the decision. Instead, the following morning, the attending physician called an ethics consultation. The chaplain (who is an ethics committee member) and the on-call ethics consult team (a subcommittee of the ethics committee) met with the physician and eventually with the family. The ethics committee consultants (a party of four—two social workers and two physicians) reviewed the chart, the patient/family history, and the conversational tradition. The medical director of the CCU was brought in to address the issues of medical futility and comfort care measures in a terminal wean. The attending physician had never been directly involved in such a procedure, which also played into his concern over physician-assisted suicide as he understood it.

A meeting of all the above and the family took place in which the following was discussed and decided:

1. Competency appeared to be a moot issue. If the patient was declared incompetent, the husband and family would become surrogate decision makers. Since they were in agreement with the

patient's decision, the decision to withdraw treatment would stand.

2. The issue of suicide was also moot since the patient hadn't voiced suicidal ideation or exhibited acute depression prior to hospitalization and had consistently complied with antidepressant medication.

3. The overall five-year survival rate given Mrs. M's multiple organ problems was less than 5 percent even had pancreatic surgery been successful.

4. The family member reiterated their total agreement with the patient's decision. They had no intention to hold anyone legally at fault. In fact, the family told the chaplain they would consider suing the doctor if he didn't comply with the patient's decision.

5. This was not physician-assisted suicide but a withdrawal of treatment based on the autonomy of a competent patient in a situation in which the benefits of further treatment were questionable.

The withdrawal of aggressive care process and the initiation of comfort care administration began, and the patient died within an hour, with her family at her bedside. Needed support was given by the chaplain and the ethics consultants to the family member in their grief, and to the attending physician as he dealt with his ethical, medical, and emotional issues connected to this case.

COMMENTARY

This is the kind of case that, in retrospect, makes one ask exactly what the problem was. There are a seeming host of possible ethical questions: the competence of the patient, the question concerning physician-assisted suicide, the "futility" of treatment, and the right of a family to refuse an ethics consultation. But most of these turned out to be somewhat peripheral to the resolution of the case. Instead, one issue took center stage. The physician was inexperienced in forgoing treatment in cases of this kind, and he suffered from a basic discomfort with the situation. One can interpret his raising of various ethical issues and his request for consultation as an attempt to sort out the source of his discomfort.

The ethics consultants cut to the heart of the matter. If the patient is competent, she has a virtually unlimited right to refuse treatment (Meisel 1992). If she lacks decision-making capacity, then her duly appointed surrogate makes the decision. In this case, either scenario would bring about the same treatment choice. It is theoretically very interesting to pursue the relationship between capacity to refuse treatment and psychological problems such as depression and suicidal ideation (Sullivan and Youngner 1994) but this issue would have had little direct import in this case. The ethics are clear, the psychological placing of responsibility for the patient's death and the clinical medical actions needed to carry out the weaning from the ventilator were less precise.

It is a legitimate function of a hospital ethics committee or ethics consultation service to review cases with which a physician is uncomfortable and to provide support of an emotional, ethical, and medical nature. This was done in this instance, i.e., a "crash course" in all aspects of forgoing treatment was provided at the bedside. However, one would suppose that it is a good idea for the physician to involve these consultants relatively early in the process rather than wait until later as in this instance. Because of the timing of the request for consultation, it seemed to the patient and family like a "stall tactic." Thus, they were initially unreceptive.

The one ethical issue that does not admit of a clear answer is whether, in a case such as this, the patient and family could refuse the ethics consultation had they persisted in that wish (Roberts, et al. 1995; Finder 1995). Obviously, they were well advised not to refuse. The consultation resulted in their wishes being respected. However, had they held firm in being uncooperative, it would seem to be their right to refuse to speak with the consultants even if the consultants continue to counsel the health-care providers.

REFERENCES

Stuart G. Finder, 1995. "Should competent patients or their families be able to refuse to allow an HEC case review? No." *HEC Forum* 7(1):51–53.

Alan Meisel, 1992. "The legal consensus about forgoing life-sustaining treatment: Its status and prospects." *Kennedy Institute of Ethics Journal* 2(4): 309–45.

Laura Weiss Roberts, Teresita McCarty, Gail Thaler, 1995. "Should competent patients or their families be able to refuse to allow an HEC case review? Yes." *HEC Forum* 7(1):48–50.

Mark D. Sullivan, Stuart J. Youngner, 1994. "Depression, competence, and the right to refuse lifesaving medical treatment." *American Journal of Psychiatry* 15(1):971–78.

Case Five:
It's the Simple Stuff: Ageism, Autonomy, and Provider Competence

KEY TERMS: *Ageism (disregard for the elderly), Narrative Ethics*

NARRATIVE

Mrs. S was a 90 year-old resident of a long-term-care facility. In addition to being about 40 pounds overweight, she had high blood pressure, diabetes mellitus, peripheral vascular disease, and was legally blind. She had frequent bowel and occasional bladder incontinence. Mrs. S was communicative and able to understand others. Her long-term memory was excellent and short-term memory only moderately impaired. She did, however, have some difficulty expressing herself verbally. She had two adult children, a son and a daughter, who lived in the area and were emotionally close to her. When they visited, they were occasionally accompanied by additional family members such as their spouses and children.

Over the course of her two-year stay at the facility, Mrs. S had become increasingly wheelchair-bound. She developed a decubitus ulcer, which was treated with topical medications and frequent washing. To relieve the constant pressure on the site, it was decided that she should not be allowed to sit up for more than two hours at a time. Her son telephoned the doctor to request that a special collagen wound dressing be applied but was told this was not necessary.

Confined to bed for long periods of time, Mrs. S became increasingly agitated and complained of pain. A nonsteroidal inflammatory agent was prescribed for the pain. Her physician also ordered the placement of an indwelling catheter so that the wound would remain dry. The son telephoned Mrs. S's physician to question this decision because Mrs. S had a previous history of urinary tract infections (UTI) and was not generally urine incontinent. The physician insisted it was important to keep the area dry and that a UTI was easily treated.

Mrs. S's condition continued to deteriorate. She complained of stomach pain and said that she could not eat. The family was puzzled about her refusal to eat, as she normally had a very hearty appetite. They asked that the doctor see the patient; he said he would see her on his next scheduled visit to the nursing home. He said he believed Mrs. S was depressed and ordered a psychiatric consult. Lorazepam, an anti-anxiety agent, was prescribed. Mrs. S continued to refuse food and gagged whenever her daughter tried to get her to eat. Although "the edge" appeared to be off her agitation, she screamed whenever she was moved or touched. The staff at the nursing home arranged for Mrs. S. to be treated at a wound-care center once a week, but the pressure sore continued to worsen. She also developed a UTI and ciprofloxacin was prescribed.

Over time, Mrs. S grew increasingly confused. This may have been due to any of a number of causes including the fact that she was confined to her bed with an indwelling catheter and had little outside stimulation. By the end of two weeks she was eating no solid food and taking only small sips of liquid. In a telephone conversation with the family, Mrs. S's physician raised the issue of inserting a feeding tube, which he assured them "was simple and not a big issue." The family was very uncertain, given their mother's precarious health and declining mental status. They did not wish to insert a tube if recovery was unlikely. The son discussed the question with his own physician as well as with a family friend who was a physician. Both suggested that it would be useful to rule out a medical condition that might be causing Mrs. S to stop eating, such as an ulcer or blockage. The family, therefore, requested a gastroscopy. Instead, Mrs. S's physician ordered a swallowing test.

A swallowing test was administered in the physical therapy department of the long-term-care facility. The therapist reported that Mrs. S had no swallowing reflex and recommended insertion of a gastric feeding tube. The family met with the social worker of the long-term-care facility to discuss the situation. She said that Mrs. S appeared to be failing and that this feeding tube might only prolong the process. She did, however, believe that Mrs. S was capable of understanding the situation and suggested she be allowed to make the final decision. The social worker assured the family that the tube could be closed and nutritional support discontinued if Mrs. S improved and began eating on her own. She also suggested that a hospice consultant was available to facilitate the discussion with Mrs. S. The son and daughter made an appointment with the hospice consultant.

When the family arrived to meet with the hospice consultant, the nurse at the desk told them the doctor had canceled the order because "Mrs. S was not at that stage yet." The family explained that they wished to meet with the consultant to discuss the pros and cons of the tube and to help ascertain Mrs. S's own wishes. When the hospice consultant arrived, the family gathered with Mrs. S to explain that her physician had recommended the gastric feeding tube because she was likely to die within a week or so since she could not eat. Repeating what they had been told by the physician, they told her that the tube would be painless. Mrs. S was unequivocal in her response—she did not want to die and agreed to the procedure. The hospice consultant restated the issues to Mrs. S, made certain that she understood, and agreed that her decision was clear.

The head nurse said Mrs. S would be scheduled for admission to a local hospital immediately because she was rapidly deteriorating from lack of nutrition. This was on the Thursday of Easter weekend. Mrs. S was not admitted to the hospital on Thursday night, as planned, because there was "no doctor available to do the procedure," i.e., insert the gastric feeding tube. Friday morning she was admitted to a different hospital. When the family arrived, they were told that a nasogastric tube, i.e., a tube that is placed through the nose, was to be inserted. They explained that their mother was supposed to have a gastric tube and would not tolerate anything going down her nose. The nurse told them no doctor was available to do the procedure because it was Easter weekend, and that if the family did not consent they would send Mrs. S back to the long-term-care facility, and she would die of lack of nutrition.

Angry and confused, the family met with the hospital's patient representative. While she was sympathetic, she said there was really nothing she could do to get a doctor to perform the procedure for which Mrs. S had been admitted. Reluctantly, the family consented to the nasogastric tube. The only physician who visited Mrs. S from Friday to Monday was the house doctor. Neither her own doctor nor the surgeon who was scheduled to insert the gastric tube saw her for three days. The nurse who examined Mrs. S before the tube insertion noted that she complained of stomach pain, but both the family and doctor attributed this to "confusion."

Mrs. S screamed during the procedure to insert the nasogastric tube, kept repeating afterward "too much pain," and pulled out the tube three times over the next two days. The third time it was not reinserted. Over the weekend Mrs. S's condition continued to deteriorate, and the family grew increasingly alarmed. She had a fever and was administered IV antibiotics for a presumed UTI. Monday morning the surgeon arrived. He expressed a reluctance to insert a tube in this patient with advanced senility but did not discuss the prognosis for a favorable outcome nor any of the possible adverse consequences of a gastric tube. The family explained that Mrs. S was able to comprehend and was unequivocal about her wish to have the tube inserted so that she might live. The surgeon performed the procedure.

THE LANGUAGE AND ISSUES OF THE CASE

The theory of informed consent versus the implementation of informed consent is at issue in this case. This is true in three ways:

1. Provider responsibility. In theory, the patient is supposed to be making the decision after receiving all the facts. The health-care providers are then supposed to carry out this decision. However, the health-care professionals and institution do not seem to be taking responsibility for aggressively pursuing the implementation of the decisions made even though they have previously agreed to them.
2. Provider competence. Even the casual reader will experience some uneasiness concerning whether the cause of Mrs. S's swallowing difficulties has been adequately pursued.
3. Respect for autonomy versus ageism. At several points in this retelling, we are left wondering whether Mrs. S's wishes and complaints are being taken as seriously as they should be.

PERSPECTIVES AND KEY POINTS OF VIEW

The Patient's Son and Daughter: These adult children faced what they considered to be a dilemma. On the one hand, they were prepared to "let their mother go" rather than prolong her pain and suffering. On the other hand, they were simply not sure that medical interventions were futile at this point. They were suspicious that their mother was not receiving completely adequate care in terms of diagnosis and treatment. They vacillated between being rather sure the care was inadequate and thinking they were imagining things due to the frustrating experiences they were having during the holiday hospitalization.

The Attending Physician: He believed that the patient's son and daughter were overreacting to everything their mother said and did. To him, she was clearly elderly and confused, and lacked the capacity to make decisions. He thought that she had a reasonable amount of life left in her and that the placement of the gastric tube was "medically indicated." When it was no longer so, he would tell the children.

The Surgeon: The surgeon was a young physician who did not think that feeding tubes should be resorted to with demented elderly patients. But since this was clearly the family's wish, he was willing to do it.

Mrs. S: Like most patients, Mrs. S wished to be made well and relieved of pain. If pain became unrelievable, she might wish to stop treatment. But she thought that she still might get better. And, besides, she wasn't always in so much pain.

POSSIBLE ALTERNATIVE ENDINGS

This is not a case that is likely to come to a simple conclusion with the aid of a skillful ethics consultant. The management of the patient's care is largely a medical issue, and the ethics consultant would be reduced to the same kind of role that the patient representative assumed when contacted.

Perhaps an additional medical opinion could be sought at some point. Similarly, when care is not delivered in a timely fashion, as in this case, families might wish to consider contacting their insurer or managed care organization (MCO). The MCO would likely be interested in extending the length of the stay, because care was not being delivered. But this patient was probably a Medicare fee-for-service enrollee, and it is just as likely that instead of seeking improved care, the MCO might focus on reducing length of stay by quickly returning the patient to the nursing home.

WHAT ACTUALLY HAPPENED

Following the procedure the surgeon met briefly with the family and told them that "by the way," he had found that Mrs. S had a duodenal ulcer. The surgeon was unavailable from that time forth. Concerned about Mrs. S's situation, the family called Mrs. S's physician several times over the next two days. Again acting on advice from friends, they asked whether she had been tested for the presence of Helicobacter pylori as a possible causative agent in the ulcer, but could not get an answer. Meanwhile the ulcer was treated with a histamine receptor agonist administered intravenously.

On the second postoperative day, Mrs. S began to improve. Nutrition was administered via the tube, which the head nurse said was a good sign because patients do not always tolerate the formula. Mrs. S was alert and responsive when awake. On the third day she was transferred back to the long-term-care facility. The family met with the health-care team and again asked if their mother had been tested for H pylori. This time they were told the results indicated the presence of H pylori and that the broad-spectrum antibiotic she was receiving was appropriate. Do-not-resuscitate orders were discussed, and the family agreed to a DNR, given their mother's complex medical situation. They asked whether it was possible that the loss of the swallowing reflex had been due to atrophy from disuse during the period of time when Mrs. S stopped eating. The physical therapist said that was possible and that if Mrs. S recovered she would be given physical therapy in an effort to restore the muscle tone.

Mrs. S continued to receive nutrition via the tube and slept most of the time. On the third day post-op, her fever rose to 105 degrees Fahrenheit. Her physician came to see her, discontinued tube feeding because he said she was developing mucous from the formula, and ordered IV fluids and a chest X ray for possible pneumonia. By 6:00 P.M. that day the family noticed a roil in Mrs. S's throat. She was extremely agitated and had a "terrified look" in her eyes. The family asked that Mrs. S be given something to calm her but was told this could not be done until after the chest X-ray.

The chest X-ray was taken at 8:00 P.M. The family waited anxiously for the results and kept asking that Mrs. S be sedated. At 10:00 P.M. the X-ray report was received by the head nurse, and the family was told the "good news" that there was no pneumonia. The nurse said they should go home. Convinced that their mother was dying, the family asked that the doctor come but was told "he had already seen Mrs. S once that day." They again asked for a sedative for Mrs. S and were told a doctor's order was required. No effort seemed to be made to obtain the order.

Mrs. S died shortly before midnight after six hours of agony for both her and her family. Her personal physician called the family at 1:00 P.M. the next day to express his condolences.

COMMENTARY

In theory, informed consent requires shared decision making in which the physician brings the medical "facts" while the patient supplies the "values" (Lidz, et al. 1988). However, a case such as this one makes clear that "moral knowing is not separable from clinical judgment" (Hunter 1996). The patient and her family have moral values that they can articulate into treatment preferences. However, their preferences depend on the medical possibilities. And, they astutely believed that these possibilities had not been completely explored.

In order to arrive at a diagnosis, the physician has to compose a story about the patient that incorporates the patient's symptoms and complaints against the backdrop of her history. But, like any composition, some are better than others. In this case, the physician was rather dismissive of the patient in general. He seems to have composed a story that was paternalistic in nature. He viewed the patient as among the demented elderly whom he would treat as he believed fit. He would justify such thinking by regarding questions—whether to place a feeding tube, whether to refer to hospice—as merely medical decisions based upon physical indications. Similarly, neither the attending physician nor the surgeon appreciated the evaluative dimension of their reasoning in dismissing the physical complaints of the patient. They believed they were being scientific while the patient was irrational and demented. Thus, they failed to see their own ageist bias in dismissing her complaints so easily. Once they were working within this narrative, it seemed to be impossible for them to see things differently (Hunter 1991, 1996). It is slightly harder to know why they were so reluctant to take the family's suggestions seriously.

One is tempted to see the health-care providers merely as incompetent and uncaring. We will not argue either for or against such an interpretation. But it is easy to see that despite the rhetoric of patient care, the health-care delivery system in question is still provider-centered rather than patient-centered. This patient's complaints were dismissed lightly and even when a satisfactory treatment plan was created, it was not implemented because it would cause inconvenience for a surgeon on a holiday. Of course, it is not obvious where to lay the blame for this. Perhaps the hospital staff members were not taking the complaint seriously enough to contact a surgeon on call. Or, perhaps a surgeon on call or the attending surgeon was coaching the staff to handle the situation this way.

So, in general, we see that respecting patient autonomy, an important principle in most ethics cases, is not an "empty" concept. This case provides several concrete examples of how the principle, if given weight in practice, would have benefited the patient and her family. Much of the problem of the case revolves around an ageist bias that prevents the physicians from understanding what is happening. And the lack of respect for autonomy is manifest in the attending physician's attitude toward shared decision making about hospice care. He is not averse to limiting aggressive treatment; he simply sees it as his decision. This forces the family members into the role of being the patient advocate. But, far and away, the issues of provider diagnostic competence and the simple kindness of the timely provision of services overshadow these moral concerns. Perhaps the models of case management that are currently evolving will bring greater scrutiny to such cases (Nash, et al. 1993) and will also enhance the physician's skills in shared end-of-life decision making (Blank 1995). It will be ironic if such oft-decried systems result in greater moral sensitivity.

REFERENCES

Linda L. Blank, 1995. "Defining and evaluating physician competence in end-of-life patient care: A matter of awareness and emphasis." *Western Journal of Medicine* 163(3):297–301.

Charles W. Lidz, Paul S. Appelbaum, Alan Meisel, 1988. "Two models of implementing informed consent." *Archives of Internal Medicine* 148:13851–89.

Michele G. Greene, Ronald Adelman, Rita Charon, Susie Hoffman 1986. "Ageism in the medical encounter: An exploratory study of the doctor-elderly patient relationship." *Language and Communication* 6(½):113–24.

Kathryn Montgomery Hunter, 1991. *Doctors' stories: The narrative structure of medical knowledge.* Princeton, NJ: Princeton University Press.

————1996. "Narrative, literature, and the clinical exercise of practical reason." *Journal of Medicine and Philosophy* 21(3):303–20.

David B. Nash, Leona E. Markson, Susan Howell, Eugene A. Hildreth, 1993. "Evaluating the competence of physicians in practice: From peer review to performance assessment." *Academic Medicine* 68(2 Suppl):S19–S22.

Advance Directives and Surrogate Decision Making

Case Six:
"But She Said She Wanted Everything"

KEY TERMS: *Advance Directives (Oral), Surrogate Decision Making, Futile Medical Treatment*

NARRATIVE

Mrs. C was a 67-year-old woman who was diagnosed as having nonresectable colon cancer six months ago. When that diagnosis was made, it was clear that the patient would eventually die but it was, understandably, not clear exactly when. This was the most recent of several admissions from a nearby nursing home for episodes of sepsis (infection) believed to be secondary to the entrance of bacteria through the friable colon cancer. On admission, the patient's general health appeared to be poor. Mrs. C looked emaciated with generalized edema (swelling) and skin excoriation (abrasions). She could not move her legs and had only gross motor movement of her upper extremities secondary to severe spinal disease. Mrs. C communicated mainly by head movements such as nodding.

The patient was given antibiotics and steroids for treatment of the sepsis and made a "full code" on the basis of discussions with her. She said that she wished to be resuscitated should the need arise. Three days after admission the patient developed acute shortness of breath, and a chest X-ray led to a differential diagnosis of congestive heart failure versus pulmonary embolism. Mrs. C also developed acute GI bleeding believed to be secondary to the colon cancer. She was admitted to the intensive care unit (ICU) for monitoring. Over the next few days, diagnostic tests gave no additional insight into the patient's condition, and Mrs. C continued to become lethargic and confused. Nevertheless, attentive patient management resulted in discharge from the ICU to a monitored unit.

The patient's mental status intermittently improved, and she complained of abdominal pain. Her pain medication was varied to see if this would further help her mental status. Over the course of several days, however, her awareness continued to decline. For much of the day, she was unconscious, and she was not oriented × 3 during her brief episodes of consciousness. This could be accounted for in several ways including possible brain metastases from the cancer. The patient also developed a pleural effusion and further malignancy was suspected.

The patient had a son who was approached regarding the use of aggressive treatment, and he requested, as had his mother, that "everything be done." She developed atrial arrhythmia, and the cardiology service was consulted. A pulmonary consultant also saw the patient and believed that she needed to be intubated and ventilated since the family wanted everything done. The consultant, however, believed Mrs. C "appeared terminal." Over the next few days aggressive vasopressor therapy was begun to try to offset the dropping blood pressure. Nevertheless, pressure continued to drop and ranged between 30 and 40 systolic on maximum vasopressor therapy. Over the next 24 hours, the patient became anuric and developed massive generalized edema. She was oozing serous fluid from her skin and other puncture sites. The patient's pupils were also fixed and dilated.

The nursing staff requested that CPR not be done if the patient arrested, because she had been hypotensive for over 48 hours. The family was reached by phone but would not consent to withholding CPR.

THE LANGUAGE AND ISSUES OF THE CASE

This case is likely to evoke cries of "futility" from the clinical staff and medical ethicists alike. If Mrs. C's heart stops beating, it is unlikely that CPR will restart it. And if the heart is successfully restarted, Mrs. C's quality of life will continue to deteriorate. The ethical reasoning behind futility cases can be easily translated into a conflict between the provider's duty to respect the patient's autonomy and his duty not to inflict unnecessary pain and suffering or indignities upon the patient. Of course, to determine whether this is truly a case where futile treatment is desired, and such duties are in conflict, we will want to know several things:

1. Was the patient competent at the time of her initial decision to be a full code?
2. Do the patient's expressed wishes apply to the situation confronting the treatment team?
3. Was the situation being adequately explained to the family in a manner that they could understand?
4. Was the family employing the correct standards of surrogate decision making? If not, what recourse is open to the health-care team?

One other point deserves mention from a medical perspective. Clearly this patient needs to be monitored closely for the potential onset of brain death. If she became brain dead, that could change what is ethically at issue.

PERSPECTIVES AND KEY POINTS OF VIEW

Mrs. C: Mrs. C's thought processes at the time of the initial conversation regarding code status are completely obscure. We have no account of how the end-of-life treatment options were presented to her or what she meant by indicating the choices she did. We are not clear how openly her impending death was discussed with her at the time of diagnosis. In general, her values and decision-making processes are the proverbial black box to us.

The Son: We do not have good insight into the motives of the patient's son, who is a central figure in this scenario. We can hypothesize that he believes he was carrying out his mother's wishes. When he said that he "wanted everything done," did he literally mean "everything" or only things that have some chance to benefit the patient?

Nursing Staff: This case was very trying for the nursing staff, especially during the final 72 hours during which the nurses described the patient as "in the process of dying." During this period, the patient was completely unresponsive and in renal failure. Her body was very swollen. Simple nursing care was very difficult because any manipulation caused skin tears. Indeed, the fact that she had "fixed and dilated pupils" suggests that she might be approaching or actually into brain death.

The nurses believed they were inflicting unnecessary pain and suffering upon the patient and began to resent the son. When the patient arrested, and they were required to start CPR, one of the nurses stated that she "just could not do chest compressions on this patient."

WHAT ACTUALLY HAPPENED

Two hours after the most recent contact with the family, who again requested that "everything be done," the patient became asystolic. (Her heart came to a standstill.) Atropine was administered, and CPR begun. Resuscitative measures were discontinued five minutes later when the attending physician was reached by phone. He gave orders to cease resuscitative efforts. The family was informed of their mother's death. They were told that CPR was tried but to no avail.

POSSIBLE ALTERNATIVE ENDINGS
AND COMMENTARY

This type of case presents severe difficulties for a treatment team. Perhaps the most revered maxim of clinical practice is "First, do no harm." Overriding this principle is usually justified by potential benefits for the patient. In this case the harms done, both in terms of physical injury and indignities perpetrated on a dying patient, were increasingly difficult to justify in terms of possible benefits.

We do not have access to the conversations between the health-care providers and the patient's son. It is difficult to know if better communication could have defused the situation. Sometimes options are presented in an open-ended fashion with the result that a family member asks for treatments that are not congruent with the goals and values they hold (Forrow 1994). When families say "Do everything possible," few mean that you should proceed with treatments that have no chance of working but guarantee further injury to the patient. By beginning the conversation with a clear articulation that the only realistic treatment goal possible is to reduce the patient's pain and suffering, the physician can often help a patient or her family to select the code status that actually will achieve this end. To begin with treatment lists is often to begin at the wrong end of the spectrum and can lead to the kind of standoff we see in this case.

The standoff might also be caused by the fact that the son simply thinks he is following the wishes of the patient. He believes the care providers are carrying out a kind of advance directive made orally by the patient. If that is the case, the health-care team can help him to explore the "substituted judgment" standard of decision making and attempt to determine what the patient would want given the current (changed) circumstances. Often, helping the family to put themselves in the patient's shoes alleviates the problem. This is especially true if they are standing on the prior statements of the patient that were made with reference to a different set of circumstances.

In a few cases, even the best communication still results in families insisting that every conceivable treatment be used. These cases are described in the literature under the heading of "futile" medical treatment or "futility." This literature is rapidly growing, and a number of senses in which the word is used have been delineated (Youngner 1988; Truog, et al. 1992). Many discussions of futility are efforts to create a new diagnostic category in which treatment no longer need be offered despite the wishes of patients and families. There is no general consensus on this issue except that perhaps we should go slowly in developing this concept lest we overlook the more common communication problems noted above and reassert paternalism in the clinical setting (Truog, et al. 1992).

Some argue that we can define a certain class of treatments as futile in the sense that they simply have been shown to have an extremely small chance of accomplishing their specific aim ("physiological futility"). Others add that futility also refers to situations that will result in an unacceptable quality of life for the patient even if the treatments accomplish their physiological aims (Schneiderman, et al. 1990; Schneiderman and Jecker 1995). Most commentators, however, believe we should restrict discussions of futility to the former category, those deemed to be "physiologically futile," and dismiss those that deal in quality-of-life considerations from this discussion (Truog, et al. 1992).

The determination that CPR will not work is generally more reliable than similar judgments with respect to other treatments. As a result, a number of respected ethicists favor not offering CPR in instances where it is physiologically futile (Blackhall 1987; Murphy 1988; Tomlinson and Brody 1990). Some hospitals have developed institutional policies that make clear that CPR need not be offered in cases where it is nearly impossible for it to be successful (Hackler and Hiller 1990; Tomlinson and Czlonka 1995; Waisel and Truog 1995; Junkerman and Schiedermeyer 1998, 28–33).

REFERENCES

Leslie J. Blackhall, 1987. "Must we always use CPR?" *New England Journal of Medicine* 317(20):1281–85.

Lachlan Forrow, 1994. "The green eggs and ham phenomena." *Hastings Center Report* 24(6):S29–S32.

J. Chris Hackler, F. Charles Hiller, 1990. "Family consent to orders not to resuscitate: Reconsidering hospital policy." *Journal of the American Medical Association* 264(10):1281–83.

Charles Junkerman, David Schiedermayer, 1998. *Practical ethics for students, interns, and residents: A short reference manual*, 2nd ed. Frederick, MD: University Publishing Group.

Donald J. Murphy, 1988. "Do-not-resuscitate orders: Time for reappraisal in long-term care institutions." *Journal of the American Medical Association* 260(14):2098–2101.

Lawrence J. Schneiderman, Nancy S. Jecker, 1995. *Wrong medicine: Doctors, patients, and futile treatment*. Baltimore, MD: Johns Hopkins University Press.

Lawrence J. Schneiderman, Nancy S. Jecker, Albert R. Jonsen, 1990. "Medical futility: Its meaning and implications." *Annals of Internal Medicine* 112(12): 949–54.

Tom Tomlinson, Howard Brody, 1990. "Futility and the ethics of resuscitation." *Journal of the American Medical Association* 264(10):1276–80.

Tom Tomlinson, Diane Czlonka, 1995. "Futility and hospital policy." *Hastings Center Report* 25(3):28–35.

Robert D. Truog, Allan S. Brett, Joel Frader, 1992. "The problem with futility." *New England Journal of Medicine* 326(23):1560–64.

David B. Waisel, Robert D. Truog, 1995. "The cardiopulmonary resuscitation-not-indicated order: Futility revisited." *Annals of Internal Medicine* 122(4): 304–8.

Stuart J. Youngner, 1988. "Who defines futility?" *Journal of the American Medical Association*, 260(14):2094–95.

Case Seven:
The Letter and Spirit of a Directive

KEY TERMS: *Advance Directives, Surrogate Decision Making, Ordinary Treatment, Forgoing Nutrition and Hydration*

NARRATIVE

An 83-year-old woman, Ms. U, was admitted to the hospital from a personal care home due to a stroke with left-sided weakness and aphasia. She had a history of Parkinson's disease, coronary artery disease, and a prior stroke several years ago. She was seen by a neurologist the day after admission who noted dysarthria (i.e., problems of speech articulation due to muscular control disturbance), a severely diminished gag reflex, and that she was not ambulatory. She did respond to right-sided commands. Speech and physical therapy were recommended.

A speech therapist also recommended that Ms. U not ingest anything by mouth due to her swallowing difficulties. A Dophoff tube (a nasogastric tube) was inserted for feedings. Ms. U subsequently pulled out the tube twice; the neurologist's notes indicated she would need a peg tube (a tube inserted into the stomach) to survive. At that time, her daughter June, who lived nearby, refused the peg tube but eventually agreed to reinsertion of the nasogastric tube as a temporary measure.

The social worker spoke at length with June. She was initially reluctant to agree to any feeding tube at all because she wanted to follow her mother's wishes as expressed in her advance directive. This living will was one of the typical forms that are used in Pennsylvania. It was so worded that Ms. U did not want artificial nutrition and hydration if she were in a terminal condition or permanently unconscious. The next day June was still uncertain and was advised to confer with her sister Donna who lived out of town. It was hoped they would clarify their mother's intent. Ms. U's family physician also spoke to June and told her that a peg tube was not an "extraordinary measure."

Due to uncertainty about the patient's decision-making capacity, a psychiatrist was consulted. He felt the patient was disoriented, lacked insight, had impairments in cognition, and was not competent to make decisions at that time. The social worker again spoke with June. June had spoken with Donna, and they were both in agreement to refuse any type of tube feeding.

During the next two days, Ms. U was seen again by the psychiatrist who found her mental status to have gradually improved to the point that she appeared to understand what a peg tube was and that it was necessary to provide her nourishment. He therefore found her to have the capacity for decision making at that time.

The hospital's ethics review group (the institution's "ethics mechanism") was summoned to review the case. It was determined that the living will was not applicable at this time and therefore could not be honored. A decision was made that members of the group would contact Ms. U's daughters to address this issue. A conference call was set up for the next morning. After the new information was presented to June and Donna, they differed on the correct decision. Time was given them so that they could speak to each other without the review group present.

In the meantime, the patient was given a barium swallow. It showed that it was still not safe for her to take nutrition orally. Due to the psychiatrist's evaluation of the patient's decision-making capacity, he referred her for a surgical consultation. The patient thought she wanted a peg tube but indicated that she wanted family agreement. Mrs. U's daughters were again contacted with this information and were presented with three options: (1) placing a Dophoff tube and physical restraints to prevent the patient from removing it, (2) placing a peg tube with no restraints, or (3) transfer of their mother to another facility for evaluation and treatment. Shortly thereafter June, who voiced opposition to artificial feeding in the conference call, called the social worker to say she agreed to insertion of the peg tube.

The peg tube was inserted the same day. Within a few days, the patient was stable and was transferred to a skilled nursing facility. Several weeks later, the ethics review group received an emotional letter from Donna. The letter showed that she was feeling guilt about her concurrence with the treatment decision. In order to help Donna understand the advance directive and the informed consent process, the social worker wrote a letter to her reviewing the decision-making process in detail. There has been no further contact from the family.

THE LANGUAGE AND ISSUES OF THE CASE

As is so often the case, the questions in this one revolve around what it means to respect the autonomy of the patient. Many of the problems concern how much information a patient's advance directive can be thought to contain and when that information should take precedence.

Clearly some members of the health-care team simply thought it was wrong to withhold nutrition and hydration from this patient. As such, they were likely to discuss this case in terms of the integrity of the medical profession, a duty of beneficence, and a duty to provide "ordinary treatment." Similarly, they would be interested in the issue of the patient's decision-making capacity. Since the interpretation of the family regarding the patient's wishes displeased the treatment team, they hoped that the patient would regain the capacity to make decisions for herself.

This case squarely raises the question whether a surrogate can make decisions for a patient in the same manner as the patient or whether the surrogate's latitude should be more restricted regarding what he or she may choose for the patient.

PERSPECTIVES AND KEY POINTS OF VIEW

Physicians and Hospital Staff: Both the attending physician and consulting physicians believed that it would be unconscionable not to "feed" the patient as she was not terminally ill. The stroke left the patient with diminished gag reflex but this need not be life threatening.

The Patient's Daughters: Both daughters wanted to honor their mother's expressed wishes and to allow her a dignified death.

The Patient: Ms. U had expressed in the advance directive that she did not want certain treatments if in a terminal state. According to the attending physician and the psychiatrist, she also seemed to express her desire to live at various points in this process.

Hospital Attorney: Looking out for the hospital's interest, the attorney believed that the patient's condition was not terminal as defined by the Pennsylvania Advance Directive for Health Care Act. Therefore, he thought that treatment should be continued.

COMMENTARY

This kind of case raises myriad questions, and there are innumerable points on which one can focus. However, it is all important to be clear on the general framework and the principles that should guide decision making in such situations. Otherwise, we run the risk of invoking legalisms as a smoke screen for one's own preferences or prejudices.

A competent patient has a virtually unlimited right to refuse treatment. A patient who lacks decision-making capacity, i.e., is incompetent, has the same rights as a competent one but the manner of exercising those rights is, of necessity, different (Meisel 1992). Usually these rights must be exercised through a written directive or through family members trying to determine what the patient would want if she possessed her decision-making capacities. These general principles must be kept in mind when dealing with such concepts as "ordinary treatment," the integrity of the medical profession, and the nuances of state laws. These concepts and regulations cannot trump a patient's fundamental rights. Rather, they are devices to assist in interpreting and respecting patient wishes.

There seems to have been little doubt in the minds of the health-care team members that Ms. U lacked capacity to make treatment decisions early in the process. Thus, her daughter(s) were appropriately contacted to act as surrogate decision makers. They made their initial assessments of the situation on the basis of their mother's advance directive. The treatment team did well to explain that the directive could not be applied in a simple deductive manner to the present case. The conditions specified by the form did not obtain. Nevertheless, the daughters are still ethically entitled to accept or refuse treatment for the patient on the basis of what they believe their mother would or would not want. The team asked them what their mother would probably say to us if she could sit up and speak. Certainly, the values that caused their mother to create an advance directive are relevant to this decision-making process even if the directive is not. The health-care team seemed to be unhappy with the decision that the daughters arrived at under such specifications. Thus, they directed attention to a variety of other issues such as legalisms surrounding the living will and questions concerning "ordinary treatment."

It became much easier to sympathize with the health-care team once Ms. U appeared to regain partial decision-making capacity. One cannot in good conscience deny life-sustaining treatment to a patient who seems to be consenting to these measures. A presumption in favor of treatment must then govern action. However, we face questions concerning whether this is a decision that the patient is making out of momentary fear, disorientation, or a desire to please the treatment team. The patient gave some indication that she wanted her daughters' agreement on this decision, and that should give the treatment team pause about their steadfast opposition to the daughters' decisions. As in case one, the team probably would have done well to bring the patient and family together for a conference on treatment goals and the particular decision at hand. This may help further to restore the patient's decision-making capacity, and it is especially appropriate in this case since the health-care team has indicated that the patient regards her daughters' opinions as having some weight in the final decision. Such a procedure requires bedside ethics consultation.

Finally, a word about misunderstandings on the part of the treatment team. We must separate motivations and reasoning. In this case the health-care team seems to be motivated by a desire to provide treatment to the patient. Like many health-care professionals, they find it very difficult to allow a patient to die who may be able to recover and who is at least semiconscious. Those involved in the case seem to have a bias in favor of administration of nutrition and hydration, and once the patient regains some consciousness, they view refusal of this treatment as "starving" the patient.

The health-care team is entitled to their feelings and, to some extent, to determinations of their standards of care. They are free to try to persuade the patient and/or her surrogate(s) to choose in accord with the judgments of the team. However, health-care professionals have an obligation to be sure that they do not give misinformation or spread misunderstanding in an effort to persuade. This happened in regard to two points:

1. **Ordinary treatment**: Legally speaking, patients have a right to refuse all treatment. It does not matter whether one calls it "ordinary" or "extraordinary." From a legal standpoint, introducing this distinction into the process was a red herring. Ethically speaking, their use of the term was also mistaken. One cannot simply call artificial nutrition and hydration "ordinary." Whether a treatment is ordinary or extraordinary depends on whether it is a measure that is "proportionate" to the case (Kelly 1991, 6–9, 13–15). That is, does it bring benefits that outweigh its burdens? In this case, the answer is not obvious. This question is exactly the point at issue between the health-care team and the patient's daughters.

2. **The Pennsylvania Advance Directive for Health Care Act**: Like the advance directive statutes of most states in the United States, this law provides immunity from liability to physicians who make a good faith effort to follow a patient's living will under specified conditions. Contrary to the inferences of the treatment team, such a law does not compel treatment under all conditions other than those it specifies (Meisel 1991, see esp. Myth 1; Meisel and Dorst 1992).

This is not to say that the particular physician or any member of the health-care team must carry out the patient's or surrogates' wishes if they personally find this a challenge to the integrity of the medical profession(s). However, if their objections are those of conscience, they should attempt transfer to other caregivers who are more willing to comply. In fairness to the team, they did present this option, but it may have been lost amid the sea of other considerations.

REFERENCES

David F. Kelly, 1991. *Critical care ethics: Treatment decisions in American hospitals.* Kansas City, MO: Sheed & Ward.

Alan Meisel, 1991. "Legal myths about terminating life support." *Archives of Internal Medicine* 151:1497–1502.

Alan Meisel, 1992. "The legal consensus about forgoing life-sustaining treatment: Its status and prospects." *Kennedy Institute of Ethics Journal* 2(4):309–45, 1992.

Alan Meisel, Stanley K. Dorst, 1992. "Living wills given life in Pa." *Pennsylvania Law Journal* XV(29):5, 29.

FOR FURTHER READING

Robert A. Pearlman, 1993. "Forgoing medical nutrition and hydration: An area for fine-tuning skills." *Journal of General Internal Medicine* 8:225–27.

Robert J. Sullivan, 1993. "Accepting death without artificial nutrition or hydration." *Journal of General Internal Medicine* 8(4):220–24.

Alan Meisel, Stanley K. Dorst, 1992. "Work in progress: Pa.'s living will law leaves unanswered question." *Pennsylvania Law Journal* XV(31):5, 10, 23.

Case Eight:
Interpreting Advance Directives:
The Problem of Partial Codes

KEY TERMS: *Informed Consent, Advance Directives, Resource Allocation (triage)*

NARRATIVE

Mr. N, an 80-year-old man, presented to the emergency department after sustaining a fall down approximately ten stairs and striking his head. Upon arrival at the ER, he was disoriented. Further evaluation revealed a large scalp laceration that was repaired. A CT scan of the head was obtained and revealed no specific evidence of head or brain injury. The patient was also noted to have a left lower lobe pneumonia that was seen on X-ray. Mr. N was admitted to a general medicine unit for further observation. The patient's code status was discussed with the family and the patient's primary care physician, Dr. Edwards. The family seemed to have a difficult time deciding but eventually came to the conclusion that Mr. N was not to be intubated or placed on a ventilator. However, all other measures were to be performed. The patient was confused and disoriented at this time and largely unable to be very helpful with this discussion.

Mr. N was found not breathing, without a pulse, and with a very slow heart rhythm early on the following morning. A "code blue" was called. The physician who responded, Dr. Dean, had not seen the patient before. Upon this physician's arrival, the patient was receiving CPR and bag-valve-mask ventilation (i.e., breathing was performed for the patient through the use of a mask and a manually operated bag). Dr. Dean attempted to intubate the patient. That is, he began to place a plastic tube into the trachea to make sure the patient could get air and to prevent him from inhaling vomitus. Dr. Dean was immediately informed of the "do not intubate" order. The patient subsequently vomited and aspirated (i.e., inhaled the vomitus). A tube was then placed in the patient's stomach to empty it.

Meanwhile, a weak pulse had returned following the administration of atropine and epinephrine, and Mr. N had a very low systolic blood pressure of 70. The patient was not breathing. Arterial blood gases on 100 percent oxygen confirmed the need for intubation in order for the patient to survive. Meanwhile, the low blood pressure responded to intravenous fluid and went to 140/70.

The patient's attending physician, Dr. Edwards, was contacted and suggested a nasal pharyngeal airway (i.e., a plastic tube through the nose to open the airway) and 100 percent oxygen. This course of action is likely to be futile if the patient is not breathing on his own. Dr. Dean felt that he was "being placed in the awkward position of being this man's executioner." He thought that placing the nasal pharyngeal airway would merely give the appearance of providing ventilatory support while he knew it would not work. Furthermore, it seemed that this recommendation was based on splitting hairs regarding what the "do not intubate" order covered.

The situation was further complicated by the fact that Dr. Dean was the only emergency department physician on duty at the time. As chance would have it, this event occurred on a busy Friday night/Saturday morning. He had been absent from the emergency department for over 20 minutes. Dean felt that leaving Mr. N could be construed as "abandonment," although nothing else could be done if the intubation was not performed. However, he could not continue to leave the emergency room unattended for much longer. Dr. Dean was caught between two dilemmas. First, he was trapped between his obligation to Mr. N and his responsibilities in the ER. And he was trapped between his responsibility to honor the wishes of the patient's surrogate (the family) and his wish to keep Mr. N from dying an unnecessary death. Dr. Dean could attempt merely to satisfy the legal requirements to treat the patient with those means not ruled out by the family but this did not satisfy his conscience.

The administrator on call was contacted and stated that he did not see a problem. He apparently felt that following the attending physician's plan was acceptable.

THE LANGUAGE AND ISSUES OF THE CASE

The major theme in this case involved balancing a respect for the wishes of the patient and family with a prudent assessment of proper medical care. Additionally, it concerns the concept of justice in the micro-allocation of resources. Put another way, how should the physician fairly distribute his time? Dr. Dean had a responsibility to this particular patient but he was also on call and had to be available to "unidentified" patients in the emergency room.

In regard to the first theme, we have a problem regarding the implementation of "partial codes" (i.e., emergency calls that require the use of some emergency procedures, such as CPR, but prohibit others, such as intubation and mechanical ventilation). The ideal of patient autonomy teaches that patients or their surrogate decision makers can choose which treatment options are appropriate and which are not. Yet this situation may have been caused by picking and choosing a combination of options that proved imprudent. Should patients or their families be able to choose treatments from a list that thereby result in partial codes?

PERSPECTIVES AND KEY POINTS OF VIEW

Dr. Edwards (patient's attending physician): Further discussion with the patient's physician revealed a line of reasoning behind the treatment choices that was not immediately evident to Dr. Dean. Mr. N had been confused prior to the event that led to his presentation to the emergency department, and this was believed to be due to senile dementia. He had also undergone a lower extremity amputation and had limited mobility. Therefore, the patient's attending physician felt that Mr. N's prognosis and potential quality of life were poor and, consequently, that he should have no "heroic" interventions, i.e., he should be a "no code." The resuscitation status of Mr. N was discussed with the family shortly after his admission to the hospital.

The family also did not wish to prolong Mr. N's suffering and thus opted not to intubate but requested performance of all other measures. Dr. Edwards felt at that time that at least preventing a prolonged stay on a ventilator prior to death would be in the patient's best interests. He thought this treatment limitation would effectively have the same results as a full no code order, and he did not wish to push the family into a decision they were not ready to make. This physician, therefore, attempted to bring about what he believed to be the appropriate outcome through sticking to the partial code during the crisis. He thought that utilizing a nasal airway and oxygen was sufficient airway management to allow Dr. Dean to feel that he was "off the hook" and still to honor the family's wishes. Dr. Edwards also thought that neither he nor Dr. Dean needed to be present at the bedside for this management.

Dr. Edwards no longer views partial codes as feasible. He also feels that such difficulties could have been avoided by beginning to discuss code status sooner with the family. If the processing and acceptance of Mr. N's condition had been begun earlier, the family would have accepted a complete no code order sooner. Dr. Edwards also believes that it is possible to direct the patient's or family's decision by the manner in which he presents the facts. Although he still believes that there are many circumstances in which it is justifiable to withhold life-sustaining treatment, he is now more cynical and paternalistic in his view of the clinical realities around this process.

Mr. N's Family: This family clearly did not want Mr. N to suffer any more than was necessary. However, when they were first asked about the use of resuscitation, many different feelings came up among the family members present at that time. In general, they were concerned about whether limiting treatment meant giving up on Mr. N. Furthermore, they had many questions about which treatments were acceptable to limit and which would be cruel or constitute euthanasia.

Dr. Dean: He also no longer believes in partial codes. This experience has made him more paternalistic in that he believes emergency physicians should have a wider latitude to override such treatment orders and intubate a patient. He reasons that the patient can always be extubated later if the family so wishes.

WHAT ACTUALLY HAPPENED

The attending physician was eventually persuaded by Dr. Dean (approximately 45 minutes into the code) to contact the family and discuss the situation. The family agreed to a complete "no code," and the patient was pronounced dead approximately 4 hours later.

COMMENTARY

This case highlights the fact that although advance directives regarding treatment limitations are no longer controversial in theory, skillful application of them in clinical practice is still a fledgling art in need of refinement. In this case there is no "advance directive" in the sense of a living will document submitted by the patient. But the directions formulated by the patient's family serve the same end: to give thoughtful instructions for application at the time of a life-threatening crisis. Like any set of directions given in anticipation of a crisis, they may not exactly fit the situation that arises and will need to be interpreted.

There is a temptation to see all advance directives as a kind of shopping list from which the patient or surrogates have selected the items they wish to buy. On this model, the customer (patient) is to be given all those things not expressly declined on the list. Hence, Dr. Dean applied the bag-valve-mask ventilation, despite the family's refusal of intubation, since the family had not specifically declined the bag-valve-mask ventilation. The bind in which this shopping list model placed the health-care providers caused them to lose faith in the process of partial treatment limitation.

The attending physician seemed to interpret the "no intubation" directive to include the manual ventilation. Perhaps this provides a clue to the unraveling of this problem. Treatment limitations are generally meant to be in the service of treatment goals (Emanuel 1991; Tomlinson and Brody 1988; Forrow 1994). The present problem seems to have arisen from confusing the treatment goals and the particular treatments. The family seemed to be clear that their general goal is to see that Mr. N's suffering not unnecessarily be increased or prolonged. But they ended up mixing and matching treatments, with the result that their attending physician felt he had to interpret their directions coyly in order that the goal be achieved.

In the short run, the family sees one major treatment goal: not increasing the patient's pain and suffering. It is odd that the result of this goal is an order to allow resuscitation efforts but not intubation. One would expect the former to contain more potential for suffering than the latter. It is the health-care provider's role to help the family to understand the way these treatments relate to the goal. In this effort, the attending physician can be fairly directive without inviting cynicism. Physicians are, after all, the experts on the particular treatments.

In sum, advance directives are not self-interpreting but must be applied on the basis of treatment goals, knowledge of the patient, and the circumstances of the situation. We should not view patient autonomy as honoring preferences for particular treatments. Patients and families should be able to trust their physician to respect their general goals and aims. Few patients and families wish to micro-manage their own care and would be happy to entrust details to their health-care providers (Churchill 1989). Physicians should keep the patient and family informed of the details and allow for their assent or dissent.

Furthermore, it is also clear that the physician's time, especially in an on-call situation such as Dr. Dean's, is a resource to be allocated in an appropriate and just manner. Dr. Dean feared "abandoning" the patient but also realized that he had a duty to other potential patients entering the ER whom he might be able to treat with greater resulting benefit. Dr. Dean seems inclined to err on the side of spending too much time with the patient-at-hand in contrast to the more typical problem, in which orders for treatment limitation lead to physician avoidance of the patient (Youngner 1987, 30). Although a "triage" approach to these problems is an established and respected view of these situations (Childress 1997, 193–213), physicians cannot be expected to make such decisions in isolation but require institutional and policy guidance in the allocation of their time and resources at the bedside (Churchill 1987, 143–47).

REFERENCES

James F. Childress, 1997. *Practical reasoning in bioethics.* Bloomington, IN: Indiana University Press.

Larry R. Churchill, 1987. *Rationing health care in America: Perceptions and principles of justice.* Notre Dame: University of Notre Dame Press.

Linda Emanuel, "The health care directive: Learning how to draft advance care documents." *Journal of the American Geriatric Society* 39(12):1221–28.

Lachlan Forrow, 1994. "The green eggs and ham phenomena." *Hastings Center Report* 24(6):S29–S32.

Tom Tomlinson, Howard Brody, 1988. "Ethics and communication in do-not-resuscitate orders." *New England Journal of Medicine* 318(1):43–46.

Stuart J. Youngner, 1987. "Do-not-resuscitate orders: No longer secret, but still a problem." *Hastings Center Report* 17(1):24–33, February 1987.

Case Nine:
When Wishes Are Not Heard

KEY TERMS: *Surrogate Decision Making, Informed Consent, Truth Telling, Conscientious Objection*

NARRATIVE

Mr. P, a 68-year-old man, went into cardiac arrest at home while watching the Steelers on television. His past medical history was significant for congestive cardiac myopathy, and he had been hospitalized on several occasions for congestive heart failure. The EMS team that arrived found Mr. P unresponsive, performed CPR, and intubated him. He was alive when brought to the emergency room with a heartbeat and very shallow but spontaneous respiration. Nevertheless, he had no response to painful stimuli. He was admitted to the intensive care unit (ICU) and placed on a respirator.

For the next several days, he remained deeply comatose and his neurological functioning was impaired. But for occasional spontaneous respiration, the patient might have been declared brain-dead. Five days into the ICU stay, Mrs. P and her two adult children told the respiratory therapist that they wished to speak to the attending physician and have all treatment discontinued except for comfort measures. Having witnessed the long course of cardiac difficulty through which they had supported Mr. P, they were convinced that he would not recover this time and that they were simply prolonging the inevitable. The physician, who had treated Mr. P for several years, discussed this with the family and indicated that he would honor their request.

Two days later, the patient's attending physician transferred Mr. P to a monitored unit where he remained on the respirator and received nutrition and hydration through a nasogastric tube. The family spent much time at the bedside motivated not only by their devotion to Mr. P, but also to "intercept" medications such as vasopressors that continued to be ordered despite their refusals. The family began to find it difficult to get in touch with the attending physician.

THE LANGUAGE AND ISSUES OF THE CASE

The issues clearly involve the rights of the family to set the treatment goals for the patient in the face of a physician whose actions indicate that he disagrees with their decision to limit treatment. The issue is complicated by the fact that the physician has not directly expressed this reluctance to the family in their conversations. So, in addition to the issue of who decides for the patient, a question of candor is involved.

Because this case represents such a classic conflict in the history of bedside medical ethics, the classic ethical terminology of medical paternalism versus the physician's duty to respect the patient's autonomy is sure to suggest itself in any discussion of this case.

PERSPECTIVES AND KEY POINTS OF VIEW

Patient's Wife and Children: They believed that they had a clear understanding of Mr. P's wishes, acquired over the long course of his illness. In their request to limit treatment, they believed that they were simply expressing Mr. P's desire not to prolong the natural process of his death. They respected the patient's attending physician, who had cared for Mr. P over the course of several years. Thus, they were extremely confused by his lack of straightforwardness and failure to comply with their wishes.

Nursing Staff: They felt caught between the proverbial "rock and a hard place." They found it difficult to understand why the physician would continue to order treatments that the family had specifically refused. The nurses identified with the plight of the family and wanted to honor their wishes but also felt a professional obligation to carry out the orders of the physician. Thus, they would carry out the treatment orders except when the family was there to refuse each intervention directly.

The Attending Physician: We do not know as much as we would like about him. We know that he had treated the patient over the course of several years, but we have only a few utterances and his actions from which to infer his motivations and feelings. On the few occasions on which a nurse would question why a specific treatment refusal was not being honored, the physician would briefly mention liability issues and then dismiss the question. We also know that he consulted the hospital's legal counsel, who told him to document the family's wishes and then to honor them. He nevertheless continued to ignore the family's wishes for several days after consulting the lawyer.

WHAT ACTUALLY HAPPENED

After seven days on the monitored floor (twelve days after admission), the family wrote a detailed letter to the doctor, which explained their position and pleaded with him to honor their refusal. To this letter, they also stapled the card of a lawyer they had placed on retainer. The physician began to honor the family's requests and withdrew all medications except those issued for palliation. He then withdrew the nasogastric tube. The patient died without being removed from the ventilator.

POSSIBLE ALTERNATIVE ENDINGS

Because the main problem in this case centered around the feelings and thoughts of the physician, which remained opaque both to the family and to us, the main alternatives involve ways of making those thoughts more transparent. In an institution in which there is an ethics committee or consultation service that facilitates communication, a call for assistance could have been made by the nursing staff, or the nurses could have presented the family with the option of initiating a consultation.

COMMENTARY

It would be easy simply to criticize the physician in this case, but that might be to miss the point. Of more interest is that we know so little about his thoughts and feelings. We can take at face value his fear of legal reprisal, but that cannot account for his behavior after consulting with the hospital's legal counsel. It is likely that the physician has some emotional, ethical, or medical objection to the withholding of treatment about which we can only speculate. Our speculations can run the gamut: perhaps he had an emotional attachment to Mr. P; he objected to extubation or withdrawal of the nasogatric tube, feeling that these actions would be "active" euthanasia; he has a religiously based "sanctity of life" philosophy. Or perhaps the physician has simply never withdrawn life-sustaining treatment from a patient before, and he is in need of mentoring through the process. (See Case 3.)

Discussions of clinical ethical issues seldom take the physician's feelings into account and thereby tend to vilify him or her in this type of situation. Although health-care professionals sometimes view ethics consultants or ethics committees as unwanted interference, it is in just this type of situation that such channels can provide an outlet for the uneasiness being experienced. Such mechanisms can provide "reality checks" to see if the physician's reactions have some factual basis that should be considered before honoring the family's wishes. They may also provide a way to allow the physician to honor his personal ethics by helping to arrange for transfer of the patient to another physician. Many hospital policies on forgoing treatment contain a "conscientious objection" clause that honors this type of personal objection (Meisel, Grenvik, et al. 1986; Miles, Singer, and Siegler 1989).

Less noble is the physician's basic avoidance of the family. Paternalism, in this era, is no longer a defensible ideal. All members of the health-care profession have some duty to truthfulness (Sheldon 1982) and to attempt to make their thinking "transparent" (Brody 1989) to those in their care. This is the only way to make informed consent and treatment refusals into meaningful ideals. Although the physician continued to treat the patient, his avoidance of the surrogate decision makers and his failure to provide adequate information regarding his actions constitutes a kind of abandonment (Katz 1984, 207–29).

REFERENCES

Howard Brody, 1989. "Transparency: Informed consent in primary care." *Hastings Center Report* 19(5):5–9.

Jay Katz, 1984. *The silent world of doctor and patient.* New York: Free Press.

Alan Meisel, Ake Grenvik, Rosa Lynn Pinkus, James V. Snyder, 1986. "Hospital guidelines for deciding about life-sustaining treatment: Dealing with health limbo." *Critical Care Medicine* 14(3):239–46.

Mark Sheldon, 1982. "Truth telling in medicine." *Journal of the American Medical Association* 247(5):651–54.

Steven H. Miles, Peter A. Singer, Mark Siegler, 1989. "Conflicts between patients' wishes to forgo treatment and the policies of health care facilities." *New England Journal of Medicine* 321(1):48–50.

Case Ten:
How Competent Need a Surrogate Be?

KEY TERMS: *Noncompliance, Surrogate Decision Making, Competence*

NARRATIVE

A 49-year-old woman, Mrs. Z, was admitted due to cardiac arrest. She was intubated and placed on a ventilator in the emergency room. Mrs. Z's history is significant for two prior cardiac arrests related to obstructive pulmonary disease secondary to heavy smoking, congestive heart failure, diabetes, obesity, hypothyroidism, and previous episodes of pneumonia. She had a long history of noncompliance with treatment plans and continued to smoke up to this most recent admission. Mrs. Z is a widow and lives with her daughter, son-in-law, and grandchildren. Her daughter and grandchildren are all believed to be mildly retarded.

After ten days on a ventilator, the attending physician suspected Mrs. Z to be brain-dead. However, a neurological consultation and EEG revealed some minimal brain activity. Nevertheless, the patient's chances of regaining consciousness or of returning to a decent quality of life seemed minimal. Given this poor prognosis, there were two treatment options. First, a skilled nursing facility that accepts ventilator-dependent patients could be sought. Or life-sustaining treatment could be limited or withdrawn, and the patient allowed to die. For instance, the patient could be extubated, and it was expected that she would die if this was done.

The patient's daughter, Nora, was approached with these options. Nora was unenthusiastic about the prospect of a nursing facility and decided, after several days, that her mother should be extubated. A final meeting with the entire health-care team was held to review this course of action, and all parties agreed upon the plan.

The following day, Mrs. Z was extubated but she continued to breathe on her own. She was transferred from the intensive care unit to a general medicine unit. The hospital social worker met with Nora to discuss nursing home placement. Nora, however, said that she thought her mother was going to die and did not want to explore the nursing home options.

THE LANGUAGE AND ISSUES OF THE CASE

The problem of the mental capacity of the surrogate decision maker clearly had the attention of the hospital staff. Thus, they are likely to discuss this case in terms of decision-making capacity. But we should ask ourselves very pointedly:

1. The social worker and the health-care team believe that a placement decision must be made. But the patient's daughter simply disagrees. Is she competent to be the surrogate decision maker?

Furthermore, one could also discuss this case in terms of justice issues, which involve using up scarce resources on patients who do not adhere to treatment regimens or healthy lifestyles.

The initial decision in this case involved how aggressively to treat this patient in the ICU. At that point, there were ethical issues raised by this patient's profile and history. For instance:

2. Can the patient's past "noncompliance" (e.g., continuing to smoke despite warnings; her obesity despite having diabetes) be considered to be expressive of a desire to die (i.e., not to be kept alive with life-sustaining technology)?
3. Even if the patient or surrogate should ask for the patient to be intubated and be a "full code," is this a fair use of expensive medical resources, given the patient's noncompliance?

PERSPECTIVES AND KEY POINTS OF VIEW

The Patient's Daughter (Nora): We have little insight into her thought processes beyond what we know from the recounting of the case. We know she believed her mother would soon die. It is not clear whether this was from a failure to appreciate the possibilities facing her or because she was relying on statements made by the physicians prior to Mrs. Z's extubation.

The Hospital Social Worker: This social worker knew from experience that patients often do not follow the most likely medical scenario. That is, prior to extubation, it seemed likely that Mrs. Z would die shortly after the removal of mechanical ventilation. However, many patients, like this one, continue to breathe on their own for quite a long time. Since the patient would no longer be receiving any of the high-tech care that requires hospitalization, the social worker believed the patient should be moved to another facility. The social worker also knew that a variety of institutional pressures would soon come to bear to make discharge of the patient imminent.

The social worker wished to avoid being too judgmental of Nora. However, from the social worker's point of view, the care plan of Mrs. Z would be much simpler and handled more expediently if some other guardian were appointed.

WHAT ACTUALLY HAPPENED

No follow-up information on this case is available.

COMMENTARY

This case has interesting aspects about it at each stage. It is initially interesting because it involves the type of patient, one typically labeled "noncompliant" in the literature, that can arouse emotional reactions from health-care professionals (Gorlin and Zucker 1983). It is, of course, the goal of medical professionalism that emotional reactions that do not contribute to the aims of the profession be dealt with appropriately rather than dominate or interfere with good patient care.

Noncompliance raises two questions in this particular case: (a) Is the lack of adherence to medical advice a direct expression of the patient's wish to die? and (b) Does a patient's prior noncompliance with care mean that it is now unjust to use expensive resources to prolong her life?

The answer to the first question is that we cannot directly find this message in the patient's actions. Smoking is an addiction, and addictions are complex phenomena. There is at least a prima facie case to be made that addictions are phenomena that defy the wishes and will of the patient rather than express them (Ferrell, Price, et. al. 1984). Although some argue that people should be held responsible for their addictive behavior in dealing with scarce commodities such as solid organs (Moss and Siegler 1991), few have made this argument in response to questions of fiscal scarcity.

The resource allocation issue is a complex one. Nevertheless, there is some evidence that smokers as a class may "pay their way" in the health-care and social service system because they tend to die younger and thereby do not consume a disproportionate share of scarce resources (Passell 1993, Barendregt et al. 1997). Furthermore, we cannot reduce this question of justice to an individual level (i.e., ask whether *this* smoker has paid her way in the system) since our concept of insurance is based on pooling risk over a class of persons, not on making each individual pay her own way. Thus, we have good reason to believe that the noncompliance question is actually a nonissue in this case.

The questions concerning the surrogate are more difficult. One must determine the competence of the daughter to make the decision for her mother. Assuming that a "sliding scale" of competence is appropriate (President's Commission 1982, 60–62; Drane 1984, 1985), we must ask if there is a clearly best decision to be made in this case and if there is a great risk to the patient from making the wrong decision. In other words, is the daughter capable of making a decision in her mother's best interest, within some reasonable construal of that term? Furthermore, how are we to assess the daughter's behavior after the extubation? There are no clear answers, but we must be careful to separate a lack of cognitive capacity or denial from a normal need for time to process a changing situation. Like any surrogate decision maker, Nora is entitled to some time, and we must not jump the gun because of our mistrust of her decision-making capacity.

Furthermore, some of the disposition problems that arise in this kind of case are relative to the structure of the particular health-care facility. For instance, if a hospital has available beds that are classified as "skilled care" or a long-term-care wing, the patient can often be transferred within the facility. This relieves the institution's concerns about reimbursement and still does not force the surrogate to transfer the patient off-site. This latter concern is important as feelings of abandonment can result from the symbolism of transporting the patient. And transferring a patient near death is simply undesirable. It may be the job of ethics committees to call such cases to the attention of those responsible for planning the design of hospital services. Clearly, making available some lower levels of care on-site can be a tremendous service to patients and families.

REFERENCES

Jan J. Barendregt, Luc Bonneux, Paul J. van der Maas, 1997. "The health care costs of smoking." *New England Journal of Medicine* 337(15):1052–57.

James F. Drane, 1984. "Competency to give informed consent." *Journal of the American Medical Association* 252(7):925–27, 1984.

James F. Drane, 1985. "The many faces of competency." *Hastings Center Report* 15(2):17–21.

Richard B. Ferrell, Trevor R. P. Price, Bernard Gert, and Bernard J. Bergen, 1984. "Volitional disability and physician attitudes toward noncompliance." *Journal of Medicine and Philosophy* 9(4):333–52.

Richard Gorlin, Howard D. Zucker, 1983. "Physicians' reactions to patients: A key to teaching humanistic medicine." *New England Journal of Medicine* 308(18):1059–63.

Alvin H. Moss, Mark Siegler, 1991. "Should alcoholics compete equally for liver transplantation?" *Journal of the American Medical Association* 265(10): 1295–97.

Peter Passell, "Experts wavering on steep rise in cigarette tax." *New York Times*, June 7, 1993, A8.

President's Commission for the Study of Ethical Problems in Medicine and Biomedical and Behavioral Research, 1982. *Making health care decisions*, Vol. 1, Washington, DC: U.S. Government Printing Office.

FOR FURTHER READING

S. Van McCrary, William L. Allen, Clarence L. Young, 1993. "Questionable competency of a surrogate decision maker under a durable power of attorney." *Journal of Clinical Ethics* 4(2):166–68.

Gail J. Povar, 1993. "Second guessing the patient's trust: Facing the challenge of the difficult surrogate." *Journal of Clinical Ethics* 4(2):168–71.

Case Eleven:
Advance Directives: Refusing Nutrition and Hydration

KEY TERMS: *Advance Directives, Surrogate Decision Making*

NARRATIVE

A 68-year-old female nursing-home resident, Ms. U, was admitted to the hospital with a fever of unknown origin (FUO), malnutrition, electrolyte imbalance, and grade IV sacral decubitus (bedsore). Her medical history is significant for a confirmed diagnosis of Alzheimer's disease. Ms. U had strong family support, and she had requested a DNR order several months before when she was a competent decision maker. Her son confirmed this request and personally wrote on her chart, "No machines for life support or feeding tubes."

The attending physician had no previous acquaintance with Ms. U. He wished to restore her nutritional status, treat the decubitus, and see if this returned her to her prior baseline health status without any further medical interventions. He therefore initiated total parenteral nutrition (TPN). He noted on the chart that the gastrointestinal (GI) route of feeding would be more appropriate in this case because of the cost factor. Each would accomplish the same goal, but a GI tube would be less costly by exponential amounts. Further, TPN would limit the ability of the hospital to discharge the patient, because the nursing home would not be able to administer this type of feeding. The physician noted in the chart that the cost–benefit ratio of TPN would make it prohibitive in the long run but that he could not force the family to accept a feeding tube. He also noted that he planned to present this case to an internal hospital board that routinely reviewed difficult cases. It was clear that the physician's main concern was to do what was ethically appropriate, but he believed that this case presented no obviously right course of action.

THE LANGUAGE AND ISSUES OF THE CASE

Much of the problem revolves around issues of withholding or withdrawing treatment and its relation to the "terminal" condition of the patient. Physicians are usually comfortable honoring requests to limit treatment when it is clear that it is being withheld for a "terminal" condition. In the case of Alzheimer's patients, a DNR order is often requested owing to the deteriorating quality of life, even though Alzheimer's is not technically a terminal illness in and of itself. Hence, at exactly what point a particularly acute and potentially treatable illness (e.g., malnutrition) should go untreated becomes a question for family consultation and clinical judgment.

PERSPECTIVES AND KEY POINTS OF VIEW

The Attending Physician: He wished to benefit the patient but wanted above all else to do the ethically appropriate thing. He approached this case with a desire to learn from it for future cases, since he was aware of the changing ethical dialogue within his hospital. As a result, he was open to consultation within the institution and had no particular agenda in treating the patient. Nevertheless, at first he felt an obligation to treat the patient because her illness seemed likely to be able to be relieved in a short period by using only a few simple treatments. Of course, he also pointed out that time might prove his assessment to be mistaken.

The Patient's Family: The family members had "come to grips" with the patient's Alzheimer's disease and did not want to see a protracted process of dying. In this desire, they also knew themselves to be expressing the wishes of their mother. Beyond these general feelings, we have little insight into their more specific assessments of the situation.

WHAT ACTUALLY HAPPENED

A week later, the hospital's review board discussed the case and recommended another conference with the family. That conference resulted in the family agreeing to a gastrostomy tube for a six-week trial period. The family members said that their views were based on their experience with their mother's former roommate at the nursing home, who had been fed for "a long time" by a tube and kept alive in a vegetative state. They hoped that this would not happen to their mother. The physician assured them that he would not continue therapy indefinitely but would continue to review the situation with them at agreed-upon intervals. The gastrotomy tube was placed, and the patient discharged to the nursing home five days later.

COMMENTARY

The case raises questions concerning the use of advance directives and DNR orders in patients who are not "terminally" ill in a narrow sense of that term. The patient suffered from Alzheimer's disease, and her consent to a DNR order in the past indicated some desire to avoid a protracted course of dying. Nevertheless, the main problem in the case stems from not knowing more specifics about her wishes, and this lack of information is again missing when we first learn of the family's refusal of a feeding tube.

DNR orders, like any treatment refusal, must be interpreted within the overall context of a patient's treatment goals (Tomlinson and Brody 1988). We do not know specifically what the patient wished to avoid by this refusal. Does she wish to die as soon as possible due to the progression of the Alzheimer's? Does she wish to avoid the indignity and pain and suffering of being resuscitated? Or is this simply a wish to avoid being technologically dependent for a protracted period at the end of her life? These same questions are raised in dealing with the family's refusal of the gastronomy tube. Advance directives or treatment refusals must be interpreted in order to answer these questions. It is this process of interpretation that the physician embarks upon through the review and consultation process.

It is particularly hard for us, as spectators, to pass judgment on the appropriate treatment goals for the patient, since we are not given much information on the patient's state of health prior to this admission (the bedsore is a somewhat troubling item). Of special interest would be to identify her previous mental status, in order to know what she might hope to return to. For instance, if the patient had been conscious and communicative prior to the onset of the FUO, it may be reasonable to think that the DNR order was not meant to apply if she could be returned to this state.

Fortunately, the family members were available to serve as the interpreters of the patient's and their own wishes. They must work with a "substituted judgment" standard and attempt to make choices for the patient as she would for herself (President's Commission 1983, 132–34; Buchanan and Brock 1989, 112–17). This standard calls for an ongoing process that keeps pace with the changing medical circumstances. In this case, the process was carried out nicely and resulted in the negotiated solution and the periodic review process that was the conclusion.

One cautionary note is in order. The attending physician in the hospital agreed to a trial period for the gastronomy tube and a review process. However, the patient was then discharged to the nursing home, where it is not clear that the hospital's attending will have influence over the course of action in the future. It would be good preventive ethics for the attending and the family to contact the appropriate persons in authority at the nursing home to be sure that this treatment plan is within the parameters of their policies and that this plan will be carried out at the nursing home. In this way, they may avoid having to "repeat procedure."

REFERENCES

Allen E. Buchanan, Dan W. Brock, 1989. *Deciding for others: The ethics of surrogate decision making*. New York: Cambridge University Press.

President's Commission for the Study of Ethical Problems in Medicine and Biomedical and Behavioral Research, 1983. *Deciding to forego life-sustaining treatment*. Washington, DC: U.S. Government Printing Office.

Tom Tomlinson, Howard Brody, 1988. "Ethics and communication in do-not-resuscitate orders." *New England Journal of Medicine* 318(1):43–46.

Case Twelve:
Does Asking Help? Problems with Pre-Hospital Advance Directives

KEY TERMS: *Advance Directives, Competence, Decision-Making Capacity, Informed Consent, Pre-hospital DNR Orders*

NARRATIVE

Mr. M, an 81-year-old man, was admitted to the emergency department because of a fainting spell, poor color, and low blood pressure. He had had coronary bypass surgery three years before and had Alzheimer's disease. He had been a resident of a nursing home for the past couple of years. Mr. M's wife was deceased, and he had one daughter who lived nearby. She was very protective and concerned regarding her father. She communicates regularly with the nursing home. Mr. M was met by his daughter upon his arrival in the emergency department, and she remained with him.

Mr. M's records from the nursing home included a document pertaining to life-sustaining measures. The staff in the medical records department had never seen this exact form before. It seemed to be an in-house record of the nursing home. As it contained no physician signature, it was not believed to be a physician's order form but a kind of advance directive. The document was signed by the daughter who indicated that in the event of a cardiac arrest or respiratory failure, cardiopulmonary resuscitation should be initiated along with the immediate transfer to a hospital. Despite the requirements of the Patient Self-Determination Act (PSDA), there was no documentation in the hospital chart that Mr. M or his daughter were asked about advance directives upon the patient's admission to the emergency room or his subsequent transfer to the medical unit.

At 10:30 P.M., Mr. M was transferred to a general medical/surgical unit from the emergency room. He was placed in a vest restraint at the request of his daughter due to his past history of intermittent bouts of night-time confusion. But, at this time, Mr. M was oriented to time and place.

About half an hour later, a nursing assessment was performed on Mr. M. It revealed him to have a dusky color and abnormal lung sounds. His chest X-ray confirmed a diagnosis of pulmonary edema (the accumulation of fluids in the lung). Respiratory care staff were notified to perform a breathing treatment to increase the patient's lung expansion and improve his ability to breathe. About one hour after admission to the medical/surgical unit, the patient's daughter came to the nursing desk and stated, "My father is having difficulty." The nurse accompanied her to the patient's bedside and was able to obtain Mr. M's vital signs. The nurse turned to the daughter and asked if she wanted her father resuscitated. The daughter said "no." Therefore, CPR was not initiated.

The patient ceased to breathe and died. At the daughter's request, an autopsy was performed to confirm the diagnosis of Alzheimer's disease.

THE LANGUAGE AND ISSUES OF THE CASE

Once again, it is easier to see what questions are likely to be fruitful in discussion than it is to find terminology in which to discuss this case. Because of the confusion regarding what Mr. M would want, terms like patient autonomy are not particularly useful. Instead we should ask certain questions:

1. What role should a particular kind of advance directive, i.e., a nursing-home directive, play in hospital treatment decisions?
2. What role should the family have in interpreting the wishes of the patient?
3. Did the patient have the capacity to make decisions? Was he incompetent because of his history of Alzheimer's disease?
4. Was it appropriate for the nurse to ask the daughter's wishes regarding cardiopulmonary resuscitation at the time of Mr. M's cardiac arrest? Was the nurse putting the daughter "on the spot"?

PERSPECTIVES AND KEY POINTS OF VIEW

The Nurse: She wasn't sure whether it would be best to resuscitate this patient. However, she thought that if she had performed cardiopulmonary resuscitation without the express permission of the patient's daughter, she could be accused of assault and battery.

The Patient's Daughter: She thought her father "had suffered enough." She had watched the Alzheimer's disease progress and hoped that when death finally came, it might be painless and easy for him. It is still not clear to the staff why the directive this daughter signed in the nursing home differed from these current wishes.

The Patient: We do not know what he thought. He seems to have been presumed to be incompetent on admission despite being oriented to time and place.

POSSIBLE ALTERNATIVE APPROACHES

Perhaps the best alternative would have been a preventive one that took place before the dilemma occurred.

1. The patient could have been asked about his wishes and the existence of any advance directive shortly after admission. The daughter could have been asked to be a party to this conversation.
2. Nursing-home staff could have been contacted after admission for any personal knowledge of the patient's wishes in addition to the conditions under which the nursing-home directive was prepared.

COMMENTARY

Fact can be stranger than fiction, and it is always more nuanced. Students who read this case too quickly sometimes characterize it as a case where the surrogate's wishes contradict the patient's advance directive. But this is a red herring. The form filled out at the nursing home cannot be taken to be the patient's advance directive, since it was signed by his daughter, not him. Most likely, the nursing home believed that Mr. M was not competent to make treatment decisions. So, they obtained instructions from his daughter. If this was the case, then the health-care providers at the hospital *may* have been justified in continuing to listen to this surrogate. Certainly, they have virtually no reason to be bound by the instructions the daughter recorded earlier in the nursing-home form.

Had the form actually been an advance directive signed by the patient that requested treatment, the hospital staff would probably have done well to treat the patient during the arrest. If they found out later that they had misinterpreted his wishes, they could then withdraw the treatment. But, if in doubt, they would have to err on the side of life (President's Commission 1983, 239–40).

But as this case stands, we cannot really sit in judgment of the actions of the nurse at the time of the patient's death. She had to act on the basis of the daughter's instructions if she felt that the daughter was appropriately exercising the patient's rights. If the nurse believed that the patient's daughter was not making a hasty decision but understood the situation and was acting according to the usual standards of surrogate decision making, then she did well not to "call a code." But if there were serious doubts that the patient's daughter understood the implications and gravity of this matter, prudence counsels erring on the side of life.

As is so often the case, we are not sure whether this patient could have spoken for himself. Of course, if he could, he should. We can sympathize with the difficulties that health-care providers face when admitting an elderly, perhaps demented, patient through the emergency room of the hospital. It is generally far less complicated at that time not to ask patients like this too many questions but to presume them to be incompetent. Of course, such a presumption is exactly the opposite of what ethics requires (Buchanan and Brock 1989: 20–23). And the general lack of solicitation regarding advance directives and the desire to formulate them is contrary to the spirit and letter of the Patient Self-Determination Act (Sabatino 1993). Unfortunately, the assumption that the patient lacked the capacity to participate in the making of directives may be all too common (Bradley, et al. 1997).

In closing, we should note that acting based upon a form poses extreme difficulty for health-care professionals. Even properly executed advance directives require a good deal of interpretation in their application to specific situations. As a result, they are often ineffectual in the highly charged emergency situation. Many states have begun to respond to this problem with the creation of pre-hospital DNR systems (Sachs, et al. 1991; Sosna, et al. 1994). These systems can provide standing physician orders regarding life-sustaining treatment for a patient who wishes them. The physician orders are then transferred with the patient from one institution to another. Of necessity, these systems must be limited in scope, and they are unlikely to solve all cases of this kind (Iserson 1995). But they are a promising direction in which to proceed to gain greater clarity for a certain subset of these situations.

REFERENCES

Elizabeth Bradley, Leslie Walker, Barbara Blechner, Terrie Wetle, 1997. "Assessing capacity to participate in discussions of advance directives in nursing homes: Findings from a study of the patient self-determination act." *Journal of the American Geriatrics Society* 45(1):79–83.

Allen E. Buchanan, Dan W. Brock, 1989. *Deciding for others: The ethics of surrogate decision making.* Cambridge: Cambridge University Press.

Kenneth V. Iserson, 1995. "If we don't learn from history. . . : Ethical failings in a new prehospital directive." *American Journal of Emergency Medicine* 13(2): 241–42.

President's Commission for the Study of Ethical Problems in Medicine and Bio-
    medical and Behavioral Research, 1983. *Deciding to forego life-sustaining
    treatment*, Washington, DC: U.S. Government Printing Office.
Charles P. Sabatino, 1993. "Surely the wizard will help us, Toto? Implementing
    the patient self-determination act." *Hastings Center Report* 23(1):12–16.
Greg A. Sachs, Steven H. Miles, Rebekah A. Levin, 1991. "Limiting resuscita-
    tion: Emerging policy in emergency medical system." *Annals of Internal
    Medicine* 114(2):151–54.
Dennis P. Sosna, Myra Christopher, Marilyn M. Pesto, David V. Morando,
    James Stoddard, 1994. "Implementation strategies for a do-not-resuscitate
    program in the prehospital setting." *Annals of Emergency Medicine* 23(5):
    1042–46.

Case Thirteen:
Advance Directives and Pregnancy

KEY TERMS: *Advance Directives, Living Wills, Surrogate Decision Making, Pregnancy, Rights of the Unborn*

NARRATIVE

Mrs. W was a 21-year-old woman who was admitted to a local hospital with shortness of breath. During this admission, she was diagnosed with PCP (pneumocystis carinii pneumonia), right parietal infarct (a blood clot in her brain) with left hemiplegia, and CMV (cytomegalovirus, an infection similar to mononucleosis). The patient was found to be HIV-positive during this admission. Her clinical condition deteriorated to the point where she was placed on intensive vasopressor therapy and antibiotics. She received maximum ventilatory support and was kept sedated all times. Despite the ventilator, she became hypoxic.

At this time, Mrs. W was 21 weeks pregnant with her second child. She had a four-year-old son. Her husband completed a palliative care sheet three weeks after admission, requesting no CPR. The patient had no previous advance directive. Mrs. W's husband recently requested that if the child should be delivered, that it not be resuscitated. An ethics consult was called by the ICU nurse in conjunction with the chief resident caring for this patient.

The patient was being cared for by the family-medicine teaching service of the hospital. Present during the consultation were the social worker, attending physician, the chief resident, the neonatologist, the patient's primary care nurse, the nursing director of the unit, the hospital attorney, and the pastoral care worker.

Under normal circumstances the family would be permitted to request the withdrawal or the withholding of life-sustaining treatments when the patient no longer could speak for herself. However the patient's pregnancy seemed to place a different light on the case, especially for the hospital attorney.

The hospital attorney contended that according to the state's living will law, all efforts must be made to provide for the birth of a viable infant. In other words, advance medical directives and the right to forgo life-sustaining treatment do not apply to pregnant women. He stated that the code status established a week ago was invalid and that the patient should be a full code until the infant becomes viable outside the mother's womb.

The social worker and primary care nurse contended that the patient's husband and son should not have to bear the consequences of the life others may choose to maintain for them. The neonatologist believed that the infant would probably reach viability by 25 weeks of gestation, but this number could be wrong by several weeks in either direction. Because he believed it would violate the patient's dignity, the resident caring for this patient did not feel he could morally "push on the woman's chest" despite the fact that she was pregnant.

THE LANGUAGE AND ISSUES OF THE CASE

In the mainstream of bioethics, a case of this type naturally suggests the usual language of a conflict between the rights, self-determination, and autonomy of a patient and her surrogate decision maker versus the paternalism of another agent. Usually such conflicts are between patient and physician; in this case it seems to be a conflict between the patient and the state. Cases involving pregnancy often evidence a contest over language. Whether we say "fetus" or "unborn child" will evidence our predisposition in resolving the case.

Several practical philosophical and legal questions quickly come to mind.

1. Does a husband have the right to make choices on the basis of what he believes would be his wife's wishes or in her best interest despite the presence of the fetus?
2. Does the hospital have the right to insist that the patient continue with all medical treatment for the next four weeks so that the child can be viable?
3. Are there rights of fetus/the unborn child?

PERSPECTIVES AND KEY POINTS OF VIEW

The Hospital Attorney: The hospital attorney very articulately discussed the legal implications for the hospital if a wrong choice was made. In his estimation, the wrong choice legally was for the hospital to agree to the moral right of the husband to withdraw life support or designate other than a full code status. He felt very confident in his opinion.

The Primary Care Nurse and the Social Worker: Both developed a professional relationship with the patient's husband and child and had much sympathy for them. They had seen the family cry at the patient's bedside and became aware of the financial burden that a chronically ill neonate would place on an already grieving family.

The Resident: He spent six weeks providing professional care to the patient and had gotten to know this woman's family. He did not feel he could morally abide by the decision to resuscitate this patient because it would be of no direct benefit and would inflict injury on her.

The Neonatologist: She was reluctant to commit to precise statements regarding the viability or lack of viability of this fetus. She agreed with the patient's physician that there was a high likelihood (greater than 80 percent) that the fetus was HIV-positive. When asked directly if this fetus could survive outside the mother's womb if labor occurred, she responded, "We have successfully resuscitated twenty-three week gestation fetuses." She would not comment upon the quality of life of these infants after resuscitation.

WHAT ACTUALLY HAPPENED

In preparation for a meeting between the ethics consultation team and the health-care team, the following preparatory steps were taken: (a) A legal opinion from outside the hospital was obtained plus (b) an ethical opinion from an ethicist at both a local children's hospital and a local neonatal unit.

A three-hour discussion took place among the ethics consultants and all the members of the treatment team. The discussion became very emotional at times. The opinions gained prior to the meeting were helpful in that they provided the consultants with valuable nonbiased information. This information helped to move the conversation away from emotional accusations and toward an intellectual discussion.

With time, the consultants were able to establish that even with CPR it was quite possible that this patient's lungs would still fail to oxygenate fully, and she would die. It was likely that CPR would be unsuccessful, if not the first time it was tried, certainly shortly thereafter. It was the opinion of the medical team that she was in danger of experiencing a respiratory arrest within a few hours. It was, therefore, the opinion of the consultants that the viability of the infant should not be of consideration at this point, since there was little chance of maintaining this woman for 24 hours even with maximum medical treatment, much less the four to five weeks recommended by the neonatologist to maintain fetal viability.

Mrs. W's code status was again made "No CPR," and she arrested ten hours later. Her husband and family were at her bedside when she died.

COMMENTARY

This case initially seemed to raise several difficult questions such as "How do we balance the rights of a pregnant woman with those of her unborn child?" "Who is responsible for the consequences of the life saved once medicine has performed its miracle?" "Just because something can be done medically does that mean it should be done?" and "If the parents cannot speak for the unborn child, then who can?" But as with most medical ethics cases, the case was resolved by recourse to the facts and not by the balancing of abstract principles.

No reasonable person or any state requires the continued performance of medical interventions that will not accomplish the physiological purpose for which they are designed. Once it was determined that this patient would die very soon no matter what medicine did, there was no reason to perform the interventions. Of course, in medicine, nothing is ever 100 percent certain, and much of the process of obtaining the "facts" was concerned with getting the physicians to render their best medical judgment. The reluctance to give such opinions is often the cause of overtreatment in the clinical setting. But physicians must not shy away from their duty to provide such opinions. Patients, families, and the health-care team must also accept these for what they are—expert opinions—and not demand infallibility.

This case would have been much more difficult to resolve if the patient could have been sustained until viability was achieved or if the fetus had already been mature enough to have a realistic chance of being delivered successfully. In that case, questions concerning the applicability of the state's living will statute would have come into play. Let us offer some guidance both from a moral and a legal perspective.

Morally speaking, it certainly seems wrong to keep a woman's body functioning against her will or the wishes of her duly designated surrogate. The principle of the sanctity of life is often honored by allowing nature "to take its course." All patients, even those who are pregnant, have a moral claim to dignity, bodily integrity, and an interest in being free of burdensome treatment. There is no moral justification for the argument that these moral considerations vanish in the face of pregnancy. Nevertheless, there is an intellectually responsible way to look at the development of life that finds viability to be an important factor in the decision-making process (Dworkin 1993).

The moral status of life, i.e., of the fetus, can be thought to increase as the contributions of nature and nurture accumulate. That is, as time goes by, nature unfolds in ever more complex ways in the individual creation, and parents and society add to this moral status by adding the effects of nurture. But this gives us relevant insight into the nature of the moral dilemma in this kind of case. The debate is not about the moral rights of the fetus but about whether the surviving family and the health-care team should be compelled to make increasing contributions to the development of this life. Given the inherent uncertainties about the relationship between the benefits of continued treatment and the corresponding burdens, the judgment of those who have the most at stake, i.e., the patient and her family, should probably be given primacy.

As a legal question, the case is probably clearer. It is clearly established that competent patients (and if incompetent, their surrogates) have the right to request the withholding or withdrawal of medical treatment even if such an act will result in their death. The protection of infants and children from abuse and neglect is also clearly expressed within both the law and ethics. However, the legal rights of the unborn are still widely debated and it is far less obvious that they can outweigh the well-established right of competent adults to be free of unwanted and burdensome medical treatment. In fact, one can raise serious questions about the constitutionality of these pregnancy exemptions in state statutes (Benton 1990; Burch 1995).

Perhaps still more important, and more disconcerting from a legal point of view, is the willingness of attorneys and health-care providers to apply provisions of advance directive statutes to patients who have no advance directive. In this case, the patient did not have a living will or a durable power of attorney for health care. But the pregnancy exemption to the state's living will law was being cited as grounds for requiring her to receive CPR. There are reasons to resist this inference.

Advance directive statutes are meant to provide immunity from civil and criminal liability to physicians who make a good faith effort to implement a patient's advance directive. Because these statutes are conferring this enormous privilege on the provider, they may require things that are not normally required in other situations. For instance, it might be better to look upon a pregnancy exemption to a living will statute as meaning that when dealing with the advance directive of a pregnant woman, the physician is not immune to the scrutiny of the justice system. Similarly, such immunity privileges are not conferred without the presence of an advance directive in the case. This does not mean the physician does something illegal. It simply means that he does not have an automatic umbrella of immunity from liability. Similarly, in trying to apply the reasoning of the advance directive statute to this case, the hospital attorney is probably trying to create an umbrella of immunity of liability for the hospital and the physician. Because one of the major conditions under which the statute takes effect is lacking, i.e., the patient has not completed an advance directive, such an attempt is probably in vain. That is, the physicians and hospital could be liable if the patient's husband brought suit against their continued treatment of her.

The complexities of this case should not mask a simple truth. Health-care providers usually fare best, both legally and morally, when they simply follow their common sense and do what seems best for their patient.

REFERENCES

Elizabeth C. Benton, 1990. "The constitutionality of pregnancy clauses in living will statutes." *Vanderbilt Law Review* 43(6):1821–37.

Timothy J. Burch, 1995. "Incubator of individual? The legal and policy deficiencies of pregnancy clauses in living will and advance health care directive statutes." *Maryland Law Review* 54(2):528–70.

Ronald Dworkin, 1993. *Life's dominion: An argument about abortion, euthanasia, and individual freedom.* New York: Alfred A. Knopf.

FOR FURTHER READING

Joel E. Frader, 1993. "Have we lost our senses? Problems with maintaining brain-dead bodies carrying fetuses." *Journal of Clinical Ethics* 4(4):347–48.

Anne D. Lederman, 1994. "A womb of my own: A moral evaluation of Ohio's treatment of pregnant patients with living wills." *Case Western Reserve Law Review* 45(1):351–77.

Janice MacAvoy-Snitzer, 1987. "Pregnancy clauses in living will statutes." *Columbia Law Review* 87(6):1280–1300.

Brendan Minogue, James E. Reagan, 1994. "Can complex legislation solve our end-of-life problems?" *Cambridge Quarterly of Healthcare Ethics* 3(1):115–24.

SECTION THREE

Discharge Dilemmas

Case Fourteen:
Negotiating Care for the Technologically Dependent Patient

KEY TERMS: *Competence, Decision-Making Capacity, Surrogate Decision Making, the Hateful or Threatening Patient, Ethical Aspects of Home Care, Placement, Disposition Issues*

NARRATIVE

Mrs. T was an 80-year-old woman who was admitted to the local hospital due to problems related to breathing: respiratory failure, CO_2 narcosis, and end-stage chronic obstructive pulmonary disease. She had a history of congestive heart failure and hyperglycemia. Mrs. T had had several previous admissions to other hospitals and during her last admission had been placed on a ventilator but was eventually weaned from it. This time, however, she was again on a ventilator, and it was doubtful that she could be removed from it.

Mrs. T was currently alert and oriented. Caregivers were able to communicate with her by "reading" her lips (she was ventilated through a tracheostomy tube so her lips were unobstructed). Mrs. T repeatedly indicated her strong desire to be able to speak and to return home. A "talking tracheostomy tube" was ordered to meet the former wish. She required total care and constant monitoring although she was able to feed herself with minimal assistance.

Mrs. T's husband was deceased. She had one daughter, Mary, with whom she lived. Mary, who was single and in her early 50s, had been recovering for a year from a motor vehicle accident in which she suffered multiple fractures. She had a history of seizure disorders and once suffered a heart attack. Mary also suffered a seizure during one visit with her mother in the hospital. She walked with a limp and used a cane to ambulate.

Mary was very verbal and aggressive in telling the physicians how to treat her mother. In particular, she had certain beliefs about which medications helped or harmed her mother, and she told the doctors what medications not to administer. The hospital staff believed that Mary had fears related to her mother's previous experiences in another hospital. Mary displayed outbursts of temper toward the residents and nursing staff, because they followed the doctor's orders despite her protests. She once threw the telephone and waggled her cane at care-givers, although these efforts did not actually seem intended to injure anyone. Mary was at times perceived as threatening and verbally abusive toward the health-care team.

Mary maintained a written diary on her mother's caregivers and the care activities. She was convinced that her mother was allergic to certain medications that the physician had prescribed. She repeatedly stated that she would not give the medications to her mother when she got her home. Mary blamed the medications for her mother's continuing deteriorating condition.

Mary was insistent that her mother would return home when discharged from the hospital. Mrs. T consistently agreed with whatever Mary said. Mary had Mrs. T's power of attorney and made it very clear that neither her mother nor she will agree to a nursing home or rehabilitation facility. "I can give my mother better care than any nursing home. I promised she would never go to a nursing home. Ain't that right, Mom?"

The social worker and other members of the health-care team met on several occasions with the patient and her daughter to discuss post-hospitalization plans. The physician was adamant that the patient needed to go to a skilled nursing home upon discharge from the hospital. At Mary's request, the social worker assisted in arranging for a home ventilator assessment with a nationally recognized durable medical equipment company. The assessment was the first step in determining the patient's suitability for the state's home ventilator program. The assessors indicated concerns regarding the electrical wiring in the home and a lack of living space since the house was quite cluttered. Additionally, the social worker had made a referral to the office of the area's agency on aging to determine what home-based services could be provided to the patient.

The home services assessment indicated that Mrs. T was eligible for skilled-care in-home nursing, but this home service would not be available because state funding for the services had been depleted and because the program was at capacity. However, a slot for limited services might soon be available and eventually full services as well. The assessor had also expressed concern regarding Mary's physical health, endurance, and ability to provide the necessary care, especially before full services were accessible.

The social worker respected the patient's will to live and her decision to return home as well as Mary's determination to respect her mother's wishes and personally to provide her with the best care possible. However, he had unanswered questions regarding Mary's motivation and strong opposition to a nursing home. There were strong ties and seemingly intertwined identities between mother and daughter. It was believed possible that Mary may have been financially motivated, since her mother's social security benefits would go to the nursing home if she were admitted there. Mrs. T had both Medicare and Medicaid insurance. The situation was also clouded by hospital personnel's suspicions that Mary may have been physically abusive toward her mother. Both Mrs. T and Mary denied any abuse. Mary felt that there was no need for the social worker to pry into her or her mother's financial situation.

The physician continued to be adamant that Mrs. T be discharged to a nursing home. The hospital's utilization review department wanted the patient to be discharged as she no longer needed medically acute care.

THE LANGUAGE AND ISSUES OF THE CASE

What should the staff do?

1. Discharge the patient to her home? Does the patient's right of self-determination override the physician's desire to keep the patient safe?
2. Keep the patient in the hospital? Is this use of acute care resources fair or just to other patients and to society? Should the staff seek a court order for placement/guardianship?

As can easily be seen from this question, there are several terms to be contested. First, the physician's and nurses' reactions toward Mary raise the question whether they are employing developed professional judgment in being suspicious of her or whether they are prejudiced toward an eccentric person of a different socioeconomic status.

PERSPECTIVES AND KEY POINTS OF VIEW

The Social Worker: The social worker had established a professional working relationship with both the patient and her daughter. The social worker had concerns about Mary's ability to provide the needed care on a 24-hour basis over a long term, and he knew of the concerns about safety reported by both the medical equipment assessment and the home service assessor. However, since options had been thoroughly and repeatedly discussed (and documented) with both Mrs. T and her daughter, the social worker believed that the autonomy of the patient had to be respected. At the same time, the health-care team needed to minimize the risks to the patient that would occur within the patient's home.

Mrs. T: We have little insight into her thought processes.

Mary (patient's daughter): As far as we know, Mary loves her mother and fears losing her. She also has been extremely stressed by the hospitalizations over the years of her mother's illness. She knows that she has been told many things by many doctors. But she knows that, in the end, she is the one who ends up caring for her mother. And she works very hard to do this by making notes about all the things she needs to remember.

The Attending Physician: He has little patience for this case. He believes that the social work staff is not acting competently. If they were, they would know that Mary is "nuts" and cannot possibly provide the kind of care at home that Mrs. T will require. He believes that, if Mrs. T is sent home, she will soon die from incompetent care, and he will be held liable.

WHAT ACTUALLY HAPPENED

After several weeks of unsuccessful attempts to wean Mrs. T off the ventilator, the physician and health-care team members met with patient and daughter to discuss discharge alternatives, risks, and benefits. These discussions took place with Mrs. T and jointly with Mrs. T and Mary. Both patient and daughter were consistently firm in their demand to discharge Mrs. T to their home. The physician yielded to the patient's wishes after documenting the events.

The social worker and respiratory therapy department again began making arrangements for Mary to be trained in ventilator care management. The staff and the medical equipment company were both involved in the education process. To comply with the concerns of all the parties involved, Mary had the wiring in the home checked by a certified electrician and provided documentation of this to the medical equipment company. After a four-month hospital stay, Mrs. T, still on a ventilator, was discharged to her home with the support of some home health services. Additional respite support services were arranged through Mrs. T's church.

To the surprise of everyone except Mary, Mrs. T was cared for at home for approximately five years until her death. On several occasions she was brought in to the emergency room for tracheostomy care. The hospital staff considered this normal even under optimal circumstances. Shortly after Mrs. T's death, Mary sent a very warm card to the social work department thanking the staff for the fine care they took of her mother and for the respect they showed in dealing with them.

COMMENTARY

This case is one of a new breed of medical ethics dilemmas. Many health-care providers will readily recognize this kind of problem, discharge dilemmas that pose conflicts between providers and the patient or family regarding long-term treatment goals. But such issues have not yet received adequate treatment within the medical ethics literature. However, this situation is rapidly changing.

Competence to give informed consent or make an informed and responsible refusal of provider recommendations is at issue in this case. On the one hand, the physician, social worker, and other members of the health-care team wish to find a suitable and safe environment for the patient. On the other hand, they do not want to misjudge the patient's ability to decide for herself and, in the name of safety, unnecessarily enforce a solution that does not respect patient autonomy. As this case makes clear, determinations of competence cannot always be done in some straightforward and formulaic way. Rather, they may involve a number of discussions to determine the adequacy of factual understanding and the stability of the expressed wishes over time.

Medical ethicists typically favor making the determination of patient and surrogate decision-making capacity relative to the risk to which the decision exposes the patient (President's Commission 1982, 60–62; Drane 1984, 1985; Buchanan and Brock 1989). That is, the higher the risk to the patient that results from the decision, the higher the standard of decision-making capacity that is invoked. In this particular case, the challenge to the health-care team is to determine exactly what the real risk is to the patient, and separate that judgment from the feelings that are created by the unorthodox and idiosyncratic nature of the decision and the decision makers.

Physicians and health-care providers, like most highly trained professionals, do not like to have their expert advice challenged. The hostility that the daughter displayed and her unorthodox beliefs regarding Mrs. T's medication can easily cause one to overstate the risks posed by their preferences. The health-care team faces the challenge of trying to understand these matters from the perspective of Mrs. T and Mary.

The health-care team, particularly the social worker, did an excellent job of determining the level of risk, exploring options to help reduce those risks while honoring the patient's wishes (the home assessments and service investigations), and negotiating certain tasks that had to be completed by Mary prior to the honoring of the patient's wishes. This provided not just a feeling that their wishes were being respected, but engendered the responsibility that was necessary to keep the patient safe at home. The social worker avoided the typical temptation that results from the risk-related standard of competence. Namely, it is easy to be overly paternalistic and label the patient incompetent when the real problem is not decision-making capacity but external risk factors (Wicclair 1990).

Although the literature on this topic is scant, a useful framework for understanding what occurred in this case is provided by analogy to the more common instance of the technologically dependent child (Lantos and Kohrman 1992). Lantos and Kohrman suggest that this type of home treatment blurs the traditional concepts, roles, and expectations of both parents and care takers. In such situations, the parents are expected to create a "mini-ICU" within their home and take on responsibilities typically delegated to hospital staff. Likewise, hospital staff are expected to give up the control they are assured within the confines of the ICU and hand it over to the parents. The focus of all of this anxiety is how best to provide for the child. There is inevitably a period of negotiation that occurs as staff and parents hammer out and adjust to their new responsibilities and decide upon a mutually preferable course of action.

In the particular case at hand, we have an adult child caring for a technologically dependent mother. But this substitution of characters does not alter the issues that Lantos and Kohrman outline, namely, the negotiation of control and responsibilities to serve the patient's best interest. This negotiation process is always stressful because it challenges the judgment of even the most self-assured family members and health-care workers.

Similarly, the issues involved in technologically dependent patients being cared for at home challenge the language of autonomy and patient wishes. In the present case, we were able to discuss and adjudicate the claims in terms of the standard autonomy model of medical decision making. But as the Lantos and Kohrman perspective makes clear, the transformation of a home into a mini-ICU is an event that involves all within a social system, not merely the patient. As a result, Nel Noddings has suggested a "response to need" perspective (Noddings 1995) rather than an autonomy and justice approach.

Finally, a word about resource allocation. It is easy in these situations to override patient autonomy and justify the transfer of the patient to the nursing home on the basis of the cost of hospitalization as these negotiations are taking place. This would have been an injustice in the long run because the in-home services better honor the patient's wishes and are probably, the most cost-effective alternative. The health-care team did not succumb to the temptation to "pass the buck" but used their facility to provide the training and procure the services that enabled them ultimately to respect the patient's wishes and reduce the total long-run cost to the health-care system. In this sense, justice and autonomy worked together because the health-care team responded to their mission to treat the patient and the family, not just the illness.

REFERENCES

Allen E. Buchanan, Dan W. Brock, 1989. *Deciding for others: The ethics of surrogate decision making*. Cambridge: Cambridge University Press.

James F. Drane, 1984. "Competency to give informed consent." *Journal of the American Medical Association* 252(7): 925–27.

James F. Drane, 1985. "The many faces of competency." *Hastings Center Report* 15(2): 17–21.

John Lantos, Arthur Kohrman, 1992. "Ethical aspects of pediatric home care." *Pediatrics* 89(5): 920–24.

Nel Noddings, 1995. "Moral obligation or moral support for high-tech home care?" In John D. Arras, ed., *Bringing the hospital home: Ethical and social implications of high-tech home care*. Baltimore, MD: The Johns Hopkins University Press, 149–65.

President's Commission for the Study of Ethical Problems in Medicine and Biomedical and Behavioral Research, 1982. *Making health care decisions*, Vol. 1, Washington, DC: U.S. Government Printing Office.

Mark R. Wicclair, 1991. "Patient decision-making capacity and risk." *Bioethics* 5(2): 91–104.

FOR FURTHER READING

John D. Arras, ed. 1995. *Bringing the hospital home: Ethical and social implications of high-tech home care*. Baltimore, MD: The Johns Hopkins University Press.

Rosalie A. Kane, Arthur L. Caplan eds. 1993. *Ethical conflicts in the management of home care: The case manager's dilemma*. New York: Springer Publishing Company.

Case Fifteen:
No Good Way Out?

KEY TERMS: *Autonomy, Elder Care, Family Autonomy, Placement, Disposition Issues, Physician-Assisted Suicide*

NARRATIVE

Mr. Y was an 80-year-old widower diagnosed with chronic obstructive pulmonary disease (COPD), probably related to many years of heavy cigarette usage. Until 11 months before, he resided with his 75-year-old wife who was diagnosed with COPD as well. They were alert and independent for most of their retirement years together. Their two children resided far away, one living about a two-hour car trip away and the other approximately eight hours travel from the family home. Both children seemed close to Mr. and Mrs. Y. They phoned weekly and would travel to be with them during periods of illness. These periods of illness and subsequent hospitalizations became more frequent. Mrs. Y's health deteriorated more rapidly, and she was eventually admitted into a nursing home. She died in this institution.

Mr. Y was hospitalized on four occasions after his wife's death for treatment of his COPD and myocardial disease. On these occasions, Mr. Y was intubated and appeared to tolerate the mechanical respirator. He was quickly weaned off the respirator each time and was able to continue living independently with the aid of home health and homemaker services.

During his third hospitalization, Mr. Y experienced episodes of confusion at night. The following day he was able to recall his losses of orientation and acknowledge them. He anticipated that once he returned home, this would no longer happen. His daughter arrived, and the hospital staff initiated discussions regarding the patient's ability to return home. The attending physician and hospital social worker were concerned about Mr. Y's ability to manage in an independent environment because of the episodes of disorientation and a diminishing strength. Various options were discussed.

Mr. Y was presented with the option of a short stay at the nursing home where his wife had resided. He agreed to a two-week stay as an intermediate step to returning to his own home. This plan was carried out, with his two children alternately staying with Mr. Y for sizable periods after his return home. Their stay with him was necessitated by the fact that Mr. Y expressed disdain for the private in-home help (nursing and housekeeping) hired by his children. Mr. Y fired these workers.

After a month at home, Mr. Y again experienced respiratory distress and was brought to the emergency room by his son. The patient was again intubated and admitted. During this admission, Mr. Y's demeanor was very different: he was alert and oriented during most of the daytime but began to display combative, agitated behavior. He would attempt to pull IV lines and remove the endotracheal tube, and even strike out at nursing staff. Furthermore, the physicians found weaning Mr. Y difficult and so continued the respiratory support.

When Mr. Y was at his most lucid, he would write to his son that he wanted the tube out. He wrote this consistently for three days and also indicated that if his heart stopped, he would not want them to try and start it again. The doctor followed the patient's orders and wrote a DNR order and weaned Mr. Y off the respirator. Mr. Y continued to breathe on his own and was transferred out of the intensive care unit (ICU). The episodes of confusion and agitation continued at night.

Discharge needs were discussed with Mr. Y and his adult children. Mr. Y refused to return to the nursing home because he felt that environment to be too restrictive. Personal care facilities were suggested by the hospital staff, and he agreed to try a facility in his town. He was at this institution for six weeks when he again began discussing with his daughter the possibility of returning to his own home. His nighttime confusion continued, and so he was encouraged to stay in the personal care facility. Mr. Y reluctantly agreed. A few days after the final conversation about returning home, Mr. Y committed suicide via ingestion of household chemicals (cleaning fluids) that he had somehow procured.

THE LANGUAGE AND ISSUES OF THE CASE

The obvious question that comes to mind involves whether the family and the professional caregivers were simply too concerned with the risks to Mr. Y of living at home and usurped his autonomy. As a result, this case is likely to be discussed in terms of respecting the patient's/resident's autonomy and delineating the line that separates beneficence from unwarranted paternalism.

In broader terms, this case raises additional questions concerning the role of the family and the role of professional caregivers.

1. To what degree are sacrifices required of adult children in order to maximize their parents' lifestyle preferences?

2. If we find that Mr. Y simply finds life burdensome and no longer wishes to continue living, what is the health-care provider's duty in helping him to meet his treatment goals (e.g., a good death)? Would aiding in such a project compromise professional integrity?

PERSPECTIVES AND KEY POINTS OF VIEW

Mr. Y's Son and Daughter: The adult children, dutiful by most standards, experienced a dilemma between giving their father control over where to live versus providing him with a safe environment. They had a strong commitment to supporting his sense of control and desire for independence. This was manifest in their willingness to stay with him for fairly long stretches of time after hospitalizations. Like most individuals, they had some limits regarding how long they were able to stay with him. Then they sought a more structured environment for him because of the dangers posed by his nightly disorientation.

After Mr. Y's suicide, the adult children seemed to make sense of it in terms of his strong desire for personal autonomy. They believed that it was in character for Mr. Y not to accept his waning control over his environment and his own mental faculties. They stated afterwards, "He always had control and the last word."

The Attending Physician: The physician was sensitive to the patient's desire for self-determination. This sensitivity could be seen in the physician's willingness to extubate Mr. Y once he could be sure that this was Mr. Y's wish. He seemed willing to follow Mr. Y's treatment limitations despite the fact that there was a great deal of "fuzziness" regarding how "terminal" the physician thought Mr. Y was at various stages.

Mr. Y: The patient's thinking and feelings are not transparent to us. It is not clear whether his suicide is prompted by his living situation, his reaction to the progressive loss of his mental faculties, or some other factor. His living situation and his disorientation are related in Mr. Y's mind as he initially attributes the disorientation to not being in his own home. It is not clear whether the patient ever came to separate these factors in his thinking and if so, which factor was foremost in Mr. Y's mind when he chose to commit suicide. Either way, it is possible that Mr. Y's suicide may express a choice that is reasonable in terms of the patient's values and his own internal standards. He had seen his wife's course of illness and her eventual death. Thus, he had firsthand experience with what he might expect in the future.

COMMENTARY

This case is something of a Rorschach test for the medical ethicist. That is, there is no clear issue that jumps out at one, but the ending is so striking that there is a temptation to use the 20/20 vision afforded by hindsight and assume that something was done that was unethical. It is not clear that anything was done wrongly; perhaps some cases will end in a tragic manner despite the best efforts of all involved. Nevertheless, it seems that we can find three questions or issues around which discussion might revolve:

1.   Was this patient's autonomy respected in the sense that he was made to feel that as long as he possessed decision-making capacity he was the final arbiter of what happened to him? That is, although the risks of living alone were clear and made it ethically acceptable for the children to try to persuade their father to leave his home, the patient still would ultimately have to decide what an acceptable risk would be. Patients/residents may have the ultimate power of choice but the actions and assessments of others may help the person to feel that he does not have any choice (President's Commission 1982, 66–68; Lidz, Fischer, and Arnold 1992).

2.   Were any other options available that were not seen at the time? For instance, could one of the children have taken Mr. Y into his or her home? Would that have helped? What was the children's duty to insure that Mr. Y had the living situation he wished?

3.   It is important not to overly medicalize the problems of the elderly. However, we should be concerned with whether a treatable depression went undiagnosed in this case (AHCPR 1993; Lyness, Noel, et al. 1997). Mr. Y's wife died less than a year earlier, and his life had been in turmoil since then. Although his actions may merely reflect normal grief and rational suicide, we are left wondering whether a treatable condition may have also been at the root of this matter (Drickamer, Lee, Ganzini 1997).

4.   Although no one would recommend that an individual clinician should actively euthanize a patient, this case is of the type that causes us, as a society, to consider the possibility of physician-assisted suicide (Quill 1991; Quell, Cassel, Meier 1992; Pence 1995, 34–47). The patient may be making a competent rational choice to take his life. Some persons question whether it is not the duty of healthcare professionals to help them do this in a humane and pain-free way rather than allow the suffering

the patient probably experienced by his own method (Miller and Brody 1995). Others argue that this would compromise the integrity of the medical profession (Kass 1991; Teno and Lynn 1991) or dehumanize us as a society (Callahan 1992). Of course, it is also possible that there are other legally and morally acceptable alternatives to assisting Mr. Y's suicide that would have still allowed him a sense of control over his death (Bernat, Gert, Mogielnicky 1993).

REFERENCES

Agency for Health Care Policy and Research (AHCPR), 1993. *Depression in primary care.* Vol. 1, *Detection and diagnosis.* Rockville, MD: Public Health Service, U.S. Department of Health and Human Services, AHCP Pub. No 93-0550.

James L. Bernat, Bernard Gert, R. Peter Mogielnicky, 1993. "Patient refusal of hydration and nutrition: An alternative to physician-assisted suicide or voluntary active euthanasia." *Archives of Internal Medicine* 153:2723–28.

Allen E. Buchanan, Dan W. Brock, 1889. *Deciding for others: The ethics of surrogate decision making,* New York: Cambridge University Press.

Daniel Callahan, 1992. "When self-determination runs amok." *Hastings Center Report* 22(2): 52–55.

Margaret A. Drickamer, Melinda A. Lee, Linda Ganzini, 1997. "Practical issues in physician-assisted suicide." *Annals of Internal Medicine* 126(2):146–51.

Leon R. Kass, 1991. "Why doctors must not kill." *Commonweal* 118(14):472–76.

Charles W. Lidz, Lynn Fischer, Robert M. Arnold, 1992. *The erosion of autonomy in long-term care.* New York: Oxford University Press.

Jeffrey M. Lyness, Tamson K. Noel, Christopher Cox, Deborah A. King, Yeates Conwell, Eric D. Caine, 1997. "Screening for depression in elderly primary care patients: A comparison of the center for epidemiologic studies Depression scale and the geriatric depression scale." *Archives of Internal Medicine* 157(4):449–54.

Franklin G. Miller, Howard Brody, 1995. "Professional integrity and physician-assisted death." *Hastings Center Report* 25(3): 8–17.

Gregory E. Pence, 1995. *Classic cases in medical ethics,* 2nd. ed. New York: McGraw-Hill.

Timothy E. Quill, 1991. "Death and dignity: A case of individualized decision making." *New England Journal of Medicine* 324(10): 691–94.

Quill, Timothy E., Christine K. Cassel, and Diane E. Meier, 1992. "Care of the hopelessly ill: Proposed clinical criteria for physician-assisted suicide." *New England Journal of Medicine* 327(19):1380–84.

Joan Teno, Joanne Lynn, 1991. "Voluntary active euthanasia: The individual case and public policy." *Journal of the American Geriatrics Society* 39:827–30.

Case Sixteen:
Family Autonomy and the Child's Best Interest

KEY TERMS: *Competence, Decision-Making Capacity, Family Autonomy ("Treating the family"), Best Interests Standard*

NARRATIVE

Betty D was a 41-year-old woman, admitted after giving birth to a 4 pound, 7 ounce son in the ambulance en route to the hospital. The baby was full-term. However, the pregnancy was unusual in that Mrs. D did not know she was pregnant until her seventh month.

Mrs. D's medical history was significant for multiple sclerosis. She stopped taking her medications when she discovered that she was seven-months pregnant. Mrs. D initially thought she was entering menopause. So, she sought no further explanation of her missed menstrual periods. She had always adhered to her medical regimen and stopped taking the medications on the advice of her physician. Prior to delivery, Mrs. D had difficulty walking but was able to do so with the aid of crutches or by holding on to objects. She was independent in her activities of daily living, and she had been able to get around town since her husband could drive.

Mr. D also had multiple sclerosis. He reportedly was not as conscientious with his medical regimen as his wife. Although confined to a wheelchair, Mr. D was able to drive a car that was modified to meet his particular needs. His driving enhanced the couple's ability to function independently in the community. Mr. D had a sister who lived in the area but with whom they kept minimal contact. There were no other nearby family members and no formal support systems. Mr. D, however, had been previously married and had a son from that marriage living in Texas.

In conversations with the nursing and social service staff, Mrs. D indicated that she wished to take the baby home but requested assistance developing child-care and parenting skills. She felt that she could manage with someone assisting her in her home three to four hours daily. Mr. D did not participate in any discussions regarding discharge planning needs but stated that he would agree to his wife's wishes. The couple's only source of income was a monthly social security disability payment, and they clearly would not be able to pay out-of-pocket for in-home services.

After giving birth, Mrs. D was hospitalized for three days. During her stay, the nursing staff raised concerns regarding her ability to care for her baby at home. Mrs. D's fine motor skills were poor, and, on several occasions, the nursing staff believed that she would have dropped the baby had they not been supervising the mother-infant interaction. At the urging of the nursing staff, the pediatrician decided that he would not discharge Baby D until 24-hour-a-day home health care was arranged.

The home-care manager from the local visiting nurse association reviewed the situation and spoke with Mrs. D. He believed that the needs of the mother and infant were too great for them to meet. It was not possible for them to provide around-the-clock services. Children and Youth Services (CYS) was asked to evaluate the situation and make specific recommendations. The agency caseworker made a home visit and subsequently met with both parents at the hospital to assess their ability to provide physical care for the infant. Weakened by complications post delivery, Mrs. D required assistance getting in and out of a chair due to her tremors. Her coordination was poor, and she seemed incapable of placing and holding a bottle in a baby's mouth. Mr. D continued to be passive throughout the home visit and did not put forward any personal preference toward the outcome of the decision-making process but simply stated "Whatever" when asked for his opinion.

Children and Youth Services decided to pursue temporary custody through the courts. Mr. and Mrs. D initially agreed with this plan but then changed their minds. Mr. D's son in Texas was also willing to take the infant. During the next several days, Mr. and Mrs. D contacted an attorney and attempted to procure discharge of the child from the hospital.

THE LANGUAGE AND ISSUES OF THE CASE

The language of this case can take several turns. One can focus on Mr. and Mrs. D and speak about the rights of the disabled and the discrimination against them that results from the societal biases. Of course, we can focus on the infant as the patient of the health-care team and emphasize their duty to look out for the interests of the child. Or we can avoid terminologically pitting the interests of the parents against those of the child by seeing the family as a unit and talk about the health-care providers' duty to "treat the family." Some questions worth exploring along each of these lines include:

1. Were the rights of the baby's mother adequately taken into account?
2. What was in the baby's best interests?
3. Should more input have been elicited from Mr. D or is this an issue that centers on the *two patients* (i.e., the baby and Mrs. D)?
4. Was family autonomy respected? Who, ultimately, was in control, the hospital staff or the parents?
5. Should the attending physician have exerted a more proactive approach in the discharge disposition of the mother and infant?
6. Were the roles played by the nursing staff and social services personnel appropriate?

PERSPECTIVES AND KEY POINTS OF VIEW

The Nursing Staff: The nursing staff were extremely concerned over the welfare of the infant, who was to enter what they felt to be a home with less-than-capable parents. It was clear that providing a safe environment in which the child would be cared for was a central concern, and the nursing staff did not think such an environment could be provided within the home. The nursing staff wished to be beneficent toward the infant and adopted an attitude of protective paternalism as their main value.

The Social Workers: This group was more sympathetic to the parents' need to have the infant in their care. The social workers solicited the involvement of Children and Youth Services originally with an eye to obtaining services to assist the parents in child care. The social workers, however, wavered in this commitment as the case progressed and were ready to go along with placement of the child.

The Parents:

(a) Mr. D. His opinions were obscured by his reticence, and it was assumed that he was not the primary decision maker in the household.

(b) Mrs. D. This mother bonded well with her child, and there was never any question of her mental and emotional fitness for motherhood. She believed that with a little outside help—i.e., the three to four hours daily that she had requested—her physical challenges in caring for the child could be ameliorated. In fact, she thought that having the care of the child as a motivating force would help her to overcome many daily obstacles of living with her illness. It was not clear at this time what she thought about her husband's role in this situation.

WHAT ACTUALLY HAPPENED

The judge refused to grant custody to Children and Youth Services. Instead, he ordered CYS to provide 24-hour sitter service for 30 days until the home situation could be adequately evaluated. The baby was discharged to his parents, who took him home. Referrals were made to the Women, Infants and Children (WIC) program and to a program that screens children regarding developmental and educational needs.

For one year, the child continued to remain in the care of his parents with in-home sitter services provided eight hours nightly. The mother was able to manage care the remaining time. CYS continued to monitor the home situation. A year after the baby's discharge, Mr. D's physical health began to decline, and he was hospitalized some distance from the family home. During this period, Mrs. D and the baby went to live with her parents. Mr. D has subsequently made some progress in his recovery, and the D's are now divorced.

POSSIBLE ALTERNATIVE ENDINGS

Trust between the family and the health-care team broke down early in this case. According to information provided in the case study, Mrs. D expressed a desire to take the baby home but requested assistance with child-care and parenting skills. The hospital staff began working with CYS to consider removal of the infant from his parents' care for safety reasons. The rationale for this action by the staff was based on beneficence that probably combined with some stereotyping of the handicapped and slipped into paternalism. Mr. and Mrs. D's strengths were not utilized in this process but an adversarial relationship developed that ended with a court decision. Possible alternative strategies could have included:

1. A multidisciplinary case conference to identify the ethical issues and differing staff viewpoints;
2. The communication process with the parents could have been stepped up. More attention to the dialogue between the parents and more explicit discussion of the best interests of all parties could have avoided an adversarial court confrontation;
3. The physicians could have taken a more proactive stance rather than let the process be driven completely by other hospital staff. Their intervention would have been especially welcomed when the situation seemed to polarize and made a court confrontation inevitable.

COMMENTARY

This case is striking as much for what is missing as for what is provided. We are provided with a narrative that is largely expressed from the point of view of the nursing staff. They see the protection of the infant's physical safety as their main responsibility. In a case in which there are at least two patients (mother and child) and a variety of interests (family autonomy, patient autonomy, the baby's need to bond with his mother, the Ds need to become competent caregivers, etc.), the nursing staff rapidly came to identify one patient and his perceived physical safety as their primary obligation. The story of Mr. and Mrs. D, while providing the backdrop for the case, vanishes into relative obscurity by the end of the case. Mr. D seems uncommunicative, and what few statements we have from Mrs. D come very early in the case. The D's are so hidden from view that their divorce comes as a complete surprise shrouded in mystery.

In the narrative that the nurses compose, the conflict is one between beneficence toward the baby and the stubbornness of the mother/parents. After some initial attempts to reach a solution that will embrace both values, these values are pitted against each other, and the nurses are on the side of the former. Once these values are conceived as in conflict, an either/or dilemma results and drives the entire case.

Mr. and Mrs. D, realizing the need to appear competent and capable in order to be seen as fit parents, put forward a united front. So, Mr. D keeps all his thoughts to himself. Their divorce suggests that there may have been a difference of opinion taking place behind the scenes or that the Ds were growing apart because of the events confronting them. Perhaps, they only felt free to air these matters after the custody battle was concluded. This couple may have had medical and support needs that were forced into hiding by opposing their rights against the "best interests" of the baby. This is usually a mistake (Nelson and Nelson 1995, 88–90).

The staff chose to place all of the emphasis on the perceived needs of the baby and thereby abdicated duties to the welfare of the parents. In doing so, the staff mentally "discharged" the parents as patients to whom they had duties and chose not to "treat the family." Clearly, compromises negotiated in a context of trust would have been preferable to this adversarial evolution. Of course, it is difficult to criticize the staff for their concerns regarding the safety of the baby. However, it is appropriate to suggest that health-care workers need to ask themselves continuously whether they "overmedicalize" problems, e.g., exaggerate risk, underestimate the capabilities of the sick, the handicapped, and the elderly, and claim that only the health-care or social welfare system is capable of solving the problems. This kind of bias often works hand-in-hand with certain stereotypes we have toward the physically challenged as well as our tendency to become melodramatic regarding the needs of infants.

Finally, in any dilemma, we must ask in which direction we should err when neither alternative seems ideal. In this case, the judge seems to have properly discerned what was at issue. That is, if we conceive the conflict to be between family autonomy and the best interest of the child, we must err toward the best interest of the child. However, unless it is clear that the family does not have the child's best interests at heart, we must assume that the child's best interest is fostered by honoring family autonomy (President's Commission 1982, 182–84; 1983, 126–29; Downie and Randall 1997).

REFERENCES

Robin S. Downie, Fiona Randall, 1997. "Parenting and the best interest of minors." *Journal of Medicine and Philosophy* 22(3):219–31.

Hilde Lindemann Nelson, James Lindemann Nelson, 1995. *The patient in the family: An ethics of medicine and families.* New York: Routledge.

President's Commission for the Study of Ethical Problems in Medicine and Biomedical and Behavioral Research, 1982. *Making health care decisions*, Vol. 1, Washington, DC: U.S. Government Printing Office.

President's Commission for the Study of Ethical Problems in Medicine and Biomedical and Behavioral Research, 1983. *Deciding to forego life-sustaining treatment.* Washington, DC: U.S. Government Printing Office.

FOR FURTHER READING

Loretta M. Kopelman, 1997. "The best-interests standard as threshold, ideal, and standard of reasonableness." *Journal of Medicine and Philosophy* 22(3): 271–89.

John D. Lantos, 1997. *Do we still need doctors?* New York: Routledge, 49–64.

The Family in Medical Decision Making

Case Seventeen:
What Does She Really Want? Coercion, Persuasion, and the Family[1]

KEY TERMS: *Autonomy, Informed Consent, Surrogate Decision-Making, The Family in Medical Decision Making*

NARRATIVE

Mrs. L was a 50-year-old woman who was transferred to this tertiary care facility from a primary care hospital. She had a husband who visited frequently, if not daily. She also had several brothers and sisters but no children. Mrs. L was currently suffering from multiple external lacerations on her hands, chest, and groin area as well as kidney failure. These health problems were related to her long-term insulin dependent diabetes. She has suffered from diabetes since childhood but the complications and consequences of this illness have increased recently with a leg amputation being necessary about a year ago. She began dialysis shortly thereafter.

Mrs. L was transferred to this tertiary care facility to have the lesions biopsied for diagnostic purposes. The lesions were open, draining, and very painful to the patient. Initial work-up ruled out vasculitis as the causal agent. Finding the source of the lesions proved difficult, and the hospitalization became prolonged as other complications developed. Mrs. L was in great pain and was placed on a sand bed and given a patient-controlled analgesia machine (PCA) to help provide relief. Despite these measures, pain continued to be a factor in the slow process of diagnostic testing.

After three weeks of hospitalization that included a variety of diagnostic tests and treatment of many complications including adjustment disorders and depressive moods, Mrs. L required surgery for perfora-

---

1. Versions of this case accompanied by variations in the commentary have been previously published in two venues: Mark G. Kuczewski, 1996. "Reconceiving the family: The process of consent in medical decision making." *Hastings Center Report* 26(2):30–37; and Mark G. Kuczewski, 1997. *Fragmentation and consensus: Communitarian and casuist bioethics*. Washington, DC: Georgetown University Press, 143–44.

tion of gastric ulcers. She was placed in the intensive care unit (ICU) postoperatively because of atrial fibrillation, and she remained intubated. After six days in the ICU, she was extubated. The patient, however, refused to be suctioned by the nursing staff after extubation. She was transferred out of the ICU ten days after her admission to that unit.

Mrs. L began to ask the nurses to stop dialysis. These requests began about two weeks into this hospitalization and continued at intervals. Each time a request was made, a discussion would be held with Mrs. L, her husband, and the attending physician. In these meetings, Mr. L would often ask Mrs. L to change her mind "for him" regarding the dialysis or other tests she was resisting. Each time, the request was granted by the patient after some resistance. On a couple of occasions, the patient agreed to further diagnostic work if her husband could be with her through the test. The nursing staff became increasingly unnerved by the situation as Mrs. L would often continue to tell the nurses that she "really" wished to stop and "just wanted to die in peace." This particular wish was always superseded by the results of the patient-husband-physician conferences.

The patient and her husband grew tired of the long hospital stay. However, neither discharge to their home nor transfer back to the primary care facility near their home was ever seriously considered as a treatment option. At one conference, it was explained to the patient that transfer to another facility might entail some of the painful diagnostic tests being repeated. This information ended all further requests for transfer.

THE LANGUAGE AND ISSUES OF THE CASE

The stability of the patient's treatment wishes is clearly at issue. Because she wavers in her statements regarding her wishes, we are not sure whether to question her decision-making capacity or to focus on possible coercion by Mr. L. Several questions are clearly on the mind of the nursing staff:

1. Which of Mrs. L's wishes are her "real" ones, e.g., what she tells the nurses or those she agrees to in conference with husband and physician?
2. Is the patient being coerced by the pressures implicit in the conference discussions or are the wishes she expresses to the nurses "off the cuff" comments that should not be taken seriously?
3. Do family members (e.g., Mr. L) have a legitimate right to have their views made a part of the treatment decisions?

4. Does the lack of diagnostic certainty mean that we should err in the direction of preserving life? Or, does the great suffering this patient has endured make her desire to stop treatment more important than the desire to diagnose and help the patient?

5. Should the lack of diagnostic certainty lead us to set a high threshold of patient competence before agreeing to terminate life-sustaining treatment?

PERSPECTIVES AND KEY POINTS OF VIEW

Mrs. L: Her views of treatment seem to vacillate somewhat depending on the degree of pain she feels, the level of optimism regarding restoration of health (i.e., relief from the lesions), and the parties she is addressing (husband or nursing staff). There is more we would like to know about her. For instance, when she asks her husband to be with her during diagnostic testing, is this because his presence makes the test bearable or because she hopes he will be persuaded by witnessing her suffering? Nevertheless, it is becoming clear that she does not find a life in the hospital, suffering greatly from the open lesions, to be valuable or acceptable.

Mr. L: He clearly loves his wife and his deep attachment to her is manifest by the amount of time he spends at her side in the hospital, including helping her through difficult and painful diagnostic tests. There is a question being raised by the nursing staff as to whether he truly has her best interest at heart or is merely serving his own interests and fear of abandonment.

The Attending Physician: The physician initially hoped to make a quick diagnosis of the lesions and provide treatment to relieve this source of pain. As such, he had little trouble during the early part of the hospital course imparting hope to the patient and her husband and counseling that withdrawal of treatment be postponed in favor of diagnostic progress. As the diagnosis proved to be elusive, the physician began to worry that he had misled the patient and her husband. He, nevertheless, feared that the patient's wishes to stop dialysis may be temporary expressions of pain that pass when she is enjoying time with her husband.

It was also an initial hypothesis of the attending physician that some of Mrs. L's statements regarding the desire to stop treatment emanated from fear of abandonment and that she made these statements to elicit commitment from her husband. However, this hypothesis dissipated with time, and the physician became increasingly concerned about how to reconcile the feelings of the patient and her husband.

The Nursing Staff: The nurses are convinced that they know that the patient "really" wishes to stop dialysis and die peacefully. The nurses believe that the physician should take the patient's statements to them as definitive of her wishes and not subject her to the "coercion" of the three-way conferences.

WHAT ACTUALLY HAPPENED

About five weeks into her hospitalization, Mrs. L remained adamant in her treatment refusals during the conference with her husband and physician. Mr. L then agreed to accept her wishes and agreed to stay by her during her death. The physician wrote a do-not-resuscitate (DNR) order and an order to discontinue dialysis. Palliative care continued to be provided. The patient died within 48 hours accompanied by her grieving husband.

POSSIBLE ALTERNATIVE ENDINGS

It is difficult to fault the course of action as it developed. A number of factors had to be balanced. It took time to be sure that little benefit could be provided to Mrs. L and that her expressions of a desire to withhold treatment were stable and abiding. Some suggestions include offering her husband psychological or other services to process his grief and also some mention to Mrs. L of alternative facilities such as hospice care that might help her to achieve her treatment goals. Furthermore, once diagnostic uncertainty prevailed, investigating transfer back to the hospital closer to home might at least have made life easier for her husband for those weeks. It is difficult to understand why the patient and her husband received such pessimistic advice when they raised the issue of transfer.

COMMENTARY

This case presents an interesting study in the concept of patient autonomy. This patient raises questions for the staff concerning her decision-making capacity as well as which statements should be considered her real wishes. Mrs. L's competence is at issue because the vacillation of her moods and wishes makes it difficult to know if her desire to cease dialysis is a fixed and abiding judgment based upon firm values. The persistence of wishes and values is an essential element of a fully competent patient (Buchanan and Brock 1989, 25).

The consensus on evaluating the capacity to consent to treatment or to refuse it emphasizes that we should set a high threshold when the risk to the patient is high and lower the standard when the risk is lower (President's Commission 1982, 60–62; Drane 1984, 1985; Buchanan and Brock 1989, 51–57). In this case, such reasoning seems to have prevailed. Early in the case, when the hope of alleviating the patient's pain was high, a higher standard was set. As the burdens of treatment became clearer and the hope of benefit faded, the patient's wish to stop treatment was taken more seriously. The physician also became convinced of the patient's firmness of opinion, and the inclination toward honoring those expressions grew.

Finally, an important question concerns what exactly is an autonomous choice. Is it one which the patient makes after deliberating by herself, or is it one made in community with the significant others that have always influenced us? Clearly, the way people test their momentary preferences and come to reflect deeply held values involves their families (Nelson and Nelson 1995, 80–81; Kuczewski 1996). But some balance must be struck between "treating the family" (Macklin 1987, 131–48; Hardwig 1990; Nelson, 1992) and submitting a vulnerable patient to familial coercion (Blustein 1993). In general, it seems as if the risk-related standard the physician employed in balancing these considerations was appropriate (Kuczewski 1996).

REFERENCES

Jeffrey Blustein, 1993. "The family in medical decisionmaking." *Hastings Center Report* 23(3):6–13.

Allen E. Buchanan, Dan W. Brock, 1989. *Deciding for others: The ethics of surrogate decision making*. New York: Cambridge University Press.

James F. Drane, 1984. "Competency to give informed consent." *Journal of the American Medical Association* 252:925–27.

James F. Drane, 1985. "The many faces of competency." *Hastings Center Report* 15(2): 17–21.

John Hardwig, 1990. "What about the family?" *Hastings Center Report* 20(2): 5–10.

Mark G. Kuczewski, 1996. "Reconceiving the family: The process of consent in medical decision making." *Hastings Center Report* 26(2):30–37.

Ruth Macklin, 1987. *Mortal choices*. Boston: Houghton Mifflin Company.

James Lindemann Nelson, 1992. "Taking families seriously." *Hastings Center Report* 22(4): 6–12.

Hilde Lindemann Nelson, James Lindemann Nelson, 1995. *The patient in the family: An ethics of medicine and families.* New York: Routledge.

President's Commission for the Study of Ethical Problems in Medicine and Biomedical and Behavioral Research, 1982. *Making health care decisions*, Vol. 1, Washington, DC: U.S. Government Printing Office.

Case Eighteen:
Withdrawing Treatment and the Family's "Returning Hero"

KEY TERMS: *Surrogate Decision Making, Substituted Judgment, Patient Autonomy, Family Autonomy*

NARRATIVE

The patient, Mrs. A, is a 72-year-old woman with Alzheimer's disease. She was transferred from a nursing home to this acute care facility because of multisystem organ failure, including congestive heart failure and impaired renal function. She also had a urinary tract infection (UTI) secondary to serratia. The patient had a long medical history and was well known at this hospital.

Mrs. A's history was significant for ongoing hypertension and a pulmonary embolism (PE) ten-years prior. Post PE, the patient had a number of cardiac and pulmonary complications which had contributed to a rapid progression of the Alzheimer's. Two years before the current admission, Mrs. A suffered a brain stem stroke with "locked in" syndrome. She was intubated and a gastrostomy tube was inserted. Mrs. A was able to understand spoken and written words. She was hospitalized for an extended period (several months) and eventually transferred to a nursing home. Physical therapists saw little, if any, rehabilitation potential in the patient.

Mrs. A had lived with her husband until the stroke two years ago. Mr. A had his own health problems. He was an insulin dependent diabetic with a lower limb amputation above the left knee. Because of his physical challenges, Mr. A realized that he could not take care of his wife and consented to the nursing-home placement. He was quite upset by this state of affairs but seemed rational in discussing the treatment issues and the appropriate course of action. A son from San Francisco, Jeremy, also arrived at the hospital and told the attending physician and staff that all decisions should come through him since his father and mother were "obviously no longer capable of handling these things." Jeremy concurred that nursing-home placement was appropriate and should be initiated.

The current hospital admission was approximately one year after that placement episode. Mrs. A was still ventilator dependent, and her mental status had deteriorated over the course of the year to the point where a preliminary diagnosis of persistent vegetative state (PVS) was made. The husband was grief stricken and agreed with the attending physician that limitations of aggressive treatment seemed appropriate. Nevertheless, Mr. A wished to speak with his minister regarding what his religion had to say on the matter. After two conferences with his minister and the hospital chaplain, Mr. A agreed that a do-not-resuscitate (DNR) order should be entered on the chart. He also began to favor withdrawal of the respirator although a final decision had not been reached when the attending physician received a call from Jeremy's attorney. The attorney stated that treatment should not be limited in any way until Jeremy arrived in town and reviewed the situation.

When Jeremy arrived, he was accompanied by his wife who was seven-months pregnant. Jeremy wished his mother to be kept alive until his wife delivered the baby so that his mother could "see her grandchild." Mr. A believed that Jeremy had "taken leave of his senses" since Mrs. A could not "see" anything and that to prolong her indignities for two additional months would serve no purpose. Nevertheless, the fear of Jeremy bringing a lawsuit temporarily froze the decision-making process.

THE LANGUAGE AND ISSUES OF THE CASE

This case initially calls to mind all of the usual terminology of end-of-life cases that we explored in Section Two. We find ourselves thinking about how to respect the patient's autonomy and wondering about what role her son's wishes have. We can clarify this scenario by asking two basic questions:

1. Who is the appropriate decision maker for Mrs. A?
2. Is Jeremy's request to delay withdrawal of treatment for his social goal (letting his mother "see" the baby), a legitimate request?

PERSPECTIVES AND KEY POINTS OF VIEW

Jeremy: It is hard to attribute a single definitive motive to him because his motivations appear to shift on the basis of different considerations. In the hospital's earlier encounter with Jeremy, he focused on making sure that his mother got all the care she might need and that the physicians paid attention to her needs. He needed to be reassured of this fact before concurring with the nursing-home placement. During the current crisis, Jeremy's motivation seems to have shifted to a particular social goal, i.e., symbolically linking this birth and death in his family. No matter what motivation, Jeremy seemed determined to play an important role in the decision-making process.

Mr. A: Mr. A was well liked by the health-care team. He was dutiful toward his wife and concerned about her well-being. He had never been very fond of Jeremy and disliked his son's domineering style. Mr. A was not very patient with Jeremy, and this resulted in little direct communication between them. In the initial case conference, Mr. A seldom addressed Jeremy directly.

The Attending Physician: He wished to see that the right thing was done but had grave concerns about trying to keep this patient alive for an additional 60 days or so. He believed that administering CPR if she arrested or doing other invasive treatments if necessary would be contrary to "what is good for her."

The Nursing Staff: They were very impressed with Mr. A and liked him a great deal. Jeremy's personal style, domineering and controlling, was offensive to them, and they wished to protect Mr. and Mrs. A from his "craziness."

WHAT ACTUALLY HAPPENED

The attending physician contacted hospital legal counsel. The lawyer told the physician that this decision could legally be made by Mr. A in concert with the physician. However, much trouble could be avoided if they could get Jeremy to concur.

After two days of conferences with Jeremy, he agreed with his father's decision to withdraw the respirator.

COMMENTARY

This case raises issues regarding the role of family members in surrogate decision making and also concerning the justice of using expensive medical resources to achieve social goals. Fortunately, the latter question, on which there is no clear ethical or legal consensus, did not have to be addressed.

The physician "treated the family" (Macklin 1987). He agreed with the hospital's legal counsel that it is better to use a small amount of additional time and resources to resolve the conflicts among family members and to head off problems, including continued conflict between Mr. A and Jeremy after Mrs. A's death. This was a great service to the family, for family members are "stuck with each other" (Nelson and Nelson 1995) and are the persons most affected by these decisions (Brock 1996).

We can say a few things that might place Jeremy's request to keep his mother alive in its proper context. The standards of surrogate decision making are clear. In serial order, we are to use the advance directive, substituted judgment, and best interest standards as applicable (Meisel 1992; Junkerman and Schiedermayer 1998, 18–19). That is, we are first to base treatment on the expressed wishes of the patient. If no wishes are known, we are to use the patient's known values, to try to think like her and do "what she would want." Finally, if the existing information about the patient's wishes and values is too sketchy, we are to base our judgment on what is in the patient's best interest. Since no clear expressions of Mrs. A's wishes are available in this narrative, we next come to the "substituted judgment" standard of surrogate decision making. It is incumbent upon Jeremy to argue that his wishes are what his mother would have wanted. Putting the decision in this perspective often enables the family member to see that he is mistaken in asserting his own rights to be the decision maker and, instead, creates empathy with the patient that can be helpful in resolving the conflict.

We can also see that this kind of case involves interpersonal dynamics. Jeremy clearly had a set of needs, such as a desire to protect his parents, that must be adequately met prior to his "letting go" of her. These needs could be met with a short period of time and conferencing with him. It is important to remember that even if there are no unusual family dynamics involved, "returning heroes" often adopt their aggressive posture because they have not been a party to the decision-making process, and they must personally repeat this process (President's Commission 1982, 126–28). This is an inconvenience to the health-care team but a ritual that is helpful to the family and preemptive of later problems.

REFERENCES

Dan W. Brock, 1996. "What is the moral authority of family members to act as surrogates for incompetent patients?" *Milbank Memorial Fund Quarterly* 74(4):599–618.

Carl Junkerman and David Schiedermayer, 1998. *Practical ethics for students, interns, and residents: A short reference manual*, 2nd ed. Frederick, MD: University Publishing Group. Original edition, 1994.

Alan Meisel, 1992. "The legal consensus about forgoing life-sustaining treatment: Its status and prospects." *Kennedy Institute of Ethics Journal* 2(4): 309–45.

Hilde Lindemann Nelson, James Lindemann Nelson, 1995. *The patient in the family: An ethics of medicine and families.* New York: Routledge.
President's Commission for the Study of Ethical Problems in Medicine and Biomedical and Behavioral Research, 1982. *Making health care decisions*, Vol. 1, Washington, DC: U.S. Government Printing Office.

FOR FURTHER READING

S. Van McCrary, William L. Allen, Clarence L. Young, 1993. "Questionable competency of a surrogate decision maker under a durable power of attorney." *Journal of Clinical Ethics* 4(2):166–68.
Gail J. Povar, 1993. "Second guessing the patient's trust: Facing the challenge of the difficult surrogate." *Journal of Clinical Ethics* 4(2):168–71.

Case Nineteen:
Families and Hope

KEY TERMS: *Family in Medical Decision Making, Competence, Decision-Making Capacity, DNR*

NARRATIVE

RQ is a 32-year-old divorced man with a diagnosis of end-stage multiple sclerosis (MS). He has two living parents and one sister. The family dynamics are dysfunctional at best, stemming from before the disease process was terminal. RQ had been living independently and had cared for his own medical needs until five years ago. As his disease progressed, he opted for an experimental drug therapy from Germany in hopes of a cure. His parents, Mr. and Mrs. Q, strongly favored this therapy and made their recommendation known to all involved. As his condition worsened, RQ had several hospitalizations and was cared for at his own home by his parents and home-care agencies.

Because his parents were such strong personalities, RQ was often not included in decision making regarding his health care. This factor also made it difficult for home-care staff and hospital caregivers to communicate effectively with the patient. Because of somewhat idiosyncratic directions and orders from the parents, the home-care staff sometimes felt compromised in the care they delivered. There were ongoing conflicts throughout the entire time RQ was cared for at home.

RQ and his parents constantly struggled among themselves for control over his care. The issue of where RQ should live was contested. He sometimes suggested he should be alone; his parents insisted he live with them. During this time, RQ wished for independence, often fighting with Mr. Q and figuratively "throwing him out" of his room. However, the reality was that, at this late stage of his illness, it was impossible for RQ to care for himself and he was dependent on his parents for help.

Early in the current hospitalization, RQ became critically ill of respiratory distress. He was quickly intubated and transferred from the medical-surgical floor to the intensive care unit (ICU). There he was placed on a ventilator. RQ would indicate to staff that he "wanted the tube out," but the physician believed that this crisis was temporary and he had a chance of remission. So, the physician and parents thought treatment should continue. No form of advance directives had been previously addressed, and no one raised the question of what to do if

112

the patient's condition deteriorated. The attending physician did not approach RQ regarding these matters because he thought that RQ was not competent to make such decisions. The consulting physicians did not know the patient well enough to participate in that discussion and left this subject to the attending.

As the hospitalization continued, RQ became more and more agitated. So, he was sedated and thereby became unable to voice his wishes. His medical condition deteriorated, and he eventually had a line inserted for hyperalimentation, a tracheostomy tube placed, and he was given a feeding tube. During this course he had several bouts of infectious processes and MRSA (Methicillin Resistant Staphylococcus Aureus) infection. As the hospitalization in the ICU continued, RQ's father became more and more controlling of his care. He would forbid his wife or RQ to have discussions with the physician, pastoral care, social service, or staff regarding future placement or the patient's code status.

As time progressed (80 days), RQ's condition stabilized. He was weaned off the ventilator. When the tracheostomy tube was plugged, RQ could speak. He initiated conversations with staff. He said that he was ready to die, that he did not ever wish to be back on "that machine," and that he wanted to go home. The family insisted that RQ be a full code and all resuscitative measures be taken. Staff became increasingly frustrated as they believed it was only a matter of time before he would need to be on mechanical ventilation.

THE LANGUAGE AND ISSUES OF THE CASE

It is difficult to know what terms with which to discuss this case. The case is prima facie one of conflict between a patient and his family members. Of course, as with many conflicts involving family members, the conflict takes place against a complex background of interdependency and care. The attending physician's assessment of RQ's decision-making capacity also means that competency is at issue. This question of capacity will need to be settled in order to make progress in resolving the case. Specifically:

1. Is this patient competent in his present condition? If so, how should his right to self-determination be protected?
2. Just how far can RQ be "self-determining"? Can he make decisions regarding placement and disposition?
3. What are the rights of the parents as his caregivers? What are the duties of the health-care team toward them? For example, can they deceive the Q's regarding code status if RQ so requests?

PERSPECTIVES AND KEY POINTS OF VIEW

The Nursing Staff and Social Work Staff: From their experience in caring for this patient for an extended period, they feel confident that they know he is now competent to make his decisions. They believe he understands and appreciates that his condition is terminal.

The Parents (Mr. and Mrs. Q): They have been caring for him for five years, and they believe they have the legal right to make his treatment decisions. They also feel he is not competent due to his illness and the effects of medication.

The Physicians: RQ has a number of physicians caring for him, and they have expressed a variety of views over the course of his treatment. They are unhappy about the prospects of having to make a choice between whose wishes to honor and would very much like the patient and his parents to come to an agreement. Some physicians feel more strongly than others about where to draw a line in the negotiating process, but in general, they evince a wait-and-see attitude.

POSSIBLE ALTERNATIVE ENDINGS

The staff did not feel they could continue to be complicit in denying the rights and wishes of a competent adult patient. In one way or another, they would have to become the patient's advocate in seeing his wishes brought to fruition. But since the patient's parents were the most important part of his social world, it was important to try to keep these familial relationships intact.

The main problem for the staff involved how to bring about a plan of care that respected the patient's rights. Some on staff wished to continue a dialogue between the family and patient simultaneously. Others on staff believed such an approach to be hopeless since the parents always managed to "drown out" RQ's opinion. They proposed creating a plan "behind the backs" of the patient's parents.

WHAT ACTUALLY HAPPENED

There were several multidisciplinary patient care conferences with physicians, nurses, social service staff, administration, and others to discuss the patient's status and discharge planning. The attending physician consulted with a psychiatrist and told the family of the consult. But the attending neglected to mention that the purpose of this psychiatric consultation was to assess RQ's capacity to make his own decisions regarding DNR status and other treatment choices. After full consultation and discussion among the attending physician, the psychiatrist, and the consulting physicians, a determination was made that this patient was competent to make decisions.

The next morning, the attending signed an order form to limit life-sustaining treatment. When the parents were informed, they were angry and hostile. They threatened to seek legal action and to remove the patient from the hospital. At this point, the hospital also sought legal advice and increased security to protect the patient from being taken from the hospital against medical advice (AMA) and also to protect the staff from any threat or risk from RQ's father.

After several days of talking to the patient and his family regarding the patient's wishes, the parents began to accept that RQ could make these decisions. Sensing that positive developments were taking place, the hospital staff began to pursue discharge planning with the patient and family. Finally, with much education, planning, and care, RQ was discharged to his parents' home. He would be cared for by his parents and home health and staff. His mother took a prehospital DNR form for use at home. When leaving the unit by ambulance, RQ thanked the staff. RQ died at home as he had wished, one week after discharge with his father and mother at his side.

COMMENTARY

This case is a quintessential one dealing with the family in medical decision making. It demonstrates how roles and identities can sometimes be intermingled and intertwined in a family unit. We believe it also shows a couple of other basic facts about families. As Hilde and Jim Nelson point out, families are stuck with each other (Nelson and Nelson 1995, 75–76). So, any solution must respect the fact that these persons still must be together. And, ultimately, the person most affected by such decisions should have the final say (Nelson and Nelson 1995, 105). In most cases, including this one, that person is the patient. These facts were considered and respected by the health-care team, and there is little that we can add to their handling of the situation.

It is interesting though to note one avenue that was not available to the treatment team. Namely, in referring to the family as "dysfunctional," one gains the hope that there can be effective treatment for them as a group. Then, once they are treated, they should be functional, and the conflicts in the case would disappear. But this is a vain hope and is not what is meant by "treating the family."

Psychotherapeutic answers to the day-to-day conflicts in the clinic are seldom possible. Instead, the health-care team ultimately had to make a moral stand. They reached a point at which the wishes and interests of the patient simply could not be ignored. The question became a matter of the method of how to respect them. For this, medical ethics has no purchase on the specific course of action to be pursued. The team simply had to take everything they knew about this family from their experience and devise the best plan they could. They seem to have calculated correctly and the interests of all were served.

REFERENCES

Hilde Lindemann Nelson, James Lindemann Nelson, 1995. *The patient in the family: An ethics of medicine and families.* New York: Routledge.

Case Twenty:
Restraints and the Family

KEY TERMS: *Physical Restraints, the Family in Medical Decision Making*

NARRATIVE

Ms. Eisen is a 55-year-old woman who has severe pulmonary hypertension with a right to left shunt. Earlier in the year, she had been living at home with nasal cannula oxygen. She had a pulmonary embolus (PE) that forced her to become dependent on high-flow face-mask oxygen. She has been rejected as a candidate for a heart/lung transplant.

She became a resident of a rather unusual type of facility, a long-term-care hospital. This is a hospital that will allow extended stays while doing diagnostic work, treatment, and rehabilitation on patients who are dependent on various technologies. The patient agreed to the use of restraints at this institution because she became disoriented at certain times. But the patient's brother did not think these measures were necessary. When Ms. Eisen got out of bed and the oxygen mask came off her face, she became hypoxic very rapidly and then fell down. She agreed to wear a posey, i.e., a vest restraint, at night, but her brother objected. He believed that the posey was curtailing her freedom.

The nursing staff had documented many episodes in which Ms. Eisen tried to get out of bed. The staff was deeply concerned that unrestricted movement of the patient would separate her from the necessary oxygen, and she would die from hypoxia. (Her oxygen saturation was pretty good with the face mask on [about 90 percent] but unrecordable without it.)

Recently Ms. Eisen became somnolent and was transferred to an acute care hospital. Her brother demanded that the sister have an attendant in the room rather than restraints. This request was honored. Ms. Eisen said she did not like having someone in the room with her all the time. An ethics consult was requested by the cardiologist and the pulmonologist who were caring for this patient.

THE LANGUAGE AND ISSUES OF THE CASE

The use of restraints normally is conceived in terms of lowering the physical risks to the patient while curtailing her freedom. So, it's normally talked about as a conflict between beneficence and respect for patient autonomy. However, in this case, the patient seemed to prefer the restraints to the alternatives her brother suggested. So, this case was likely to be seen as a conflict between family members (assuming the patient possessed decision-making capacity). Some practical questions include the following:

1. How much voice in the use of an intervention, e.g., restraints, should a family have when the patient seemingly possesses decision-making capacities of her own?
2. What long-term-care strategies should be devised for a patient who requires a high level of care in order to be kept safe while allowing her discharge from the acute care hospital?
3. Is the use of restraints appropriate in this case?

PERSPECTIVES AND KEY POINTS OF VIEW

Nursing Staff: The nursing staff is aware that the oxygen is necessary for the life of the patient. It is unclear exactly what happens at night, i.e., whether Ms. Eisen's movements knocked the mask off or if her movements made her hypoxic, panic-stricken, and unable to think clearly about maintaining the face mask in position. The staff believes a posey would help decrease the incidence of mask removal, whatever the cause. They are arguing that the posey should not be perceived as a limitation, but rather a reminder of the need to be cautious.

Ms. Eisen (the patient): The patient stated to health-care providers that a posey overnight was acceptable and that having someone in her room all the time was not. The health-care providers have not questioned the patient's decision-making capacity and believe that she was expressing her true preferences.

The Patient's Brother: The brother interpreted the restraints as limiting the patient's freedom. Being restrained, he believes, caused his sister to become agitated and to struggle, which increased her need for oxygen. This increased need may not be met and the resultant hypoxia precipitated the inappropriate behavior of getting up out of bed and away from the oxygen.

WHAT ACTUALLY HAPPENED

An ethics committee reviewed the case. Three issues were discussed. First, the committee members were concerned that Ms. Eisen's brother was making patient-care decisions when no one had declared the patient to lack decision-making capacity. It was suggested that the patient, the brother, and the staff meet to review care options so that all three would hear each other's concerns. Since the patient was thought to possess decision-making capacity, if conflict persisted, the patient should choose her course of therapy.

The second concern was the long-term care of this patient. She was not a transplant candidate, which is the only hope for cure. The patient understood this, but insisted upon being resuscitated should she go into cardiac arrest. Thus, she could not be a hospice candidate. At the time of the ethics committee meeting, the patient was stable and did not need the services of the acute care hospital. The pulmonary embolus was slow to resolve and forced a higher level of nursing care than was available at local nursing homes. This patient was turned down for readmittance to the long-term-care hospital because of the discrepancies between her and her brother about the use of restraints. It was hoped the planned conference would help to define specific treatment plans and possibly make discharge to that facility an option.

The third issue was that of the use of restraints on Ms. Eisen. There was documentation that the patient's night movements shifted her beyond the reach of the oxygen tubing, which was literally sustaining life at this time. Therefore it seemed reasonable to use a restraint to remind her that she must not stray from the mask. She was bedridden and any effort such as sitting up made her hypoxic.

The ethics committee recommended that the patient, her brother, and the health-care team have a conversation about the issue of restraints. The health-care team should thoroughly explain the reasons for the use of restraints. It was clear that Ms. Eisen accepted her brother as part of her support system during her illness, but he did not understand that as long as she was deemed to possess decision-making capacity, her wishes must be honored. They needed to listen to each other's concerns about each system of restraint and try to reach an agreement acceptable to both of them and the staff, with the first priority given to the patient.

The outcome of the discussions was that the patient's brother gained a greater appreciation of her desire for privacy in her room at night. It was decided that when he came to visit and could stay overnight, he could act as the observer. But this would likely be infrequent. Most nights, the patient would wear the posey. However, the health-care team helped to devise an alternating system of posey at night with a hired observer during the day so that Ms. Eisen would not be restrained constantly. When visitors who were willing to take on the responsibility of "observant restraint" were present, the hospital attendant could leave, and Ms. Eisen could have some privacy. This system was also likely to be acceptable to a long-term-care hospital or even to some more technologically oriented nursing homes. So, the hospital social worker began to seek discharge options for the patient.

Ms. Eisen did not have an advance directive, and the ethics consultants pointed out that this would be a good time for her to complete one. The use of restraints was addressed in the directive. This directive would be useful to the long-term-care facility in the event that the patient lost her decision-making capacity.

COMMENTARY

Restraints have been used in hospitals, nursing homes, and psychiatric settings for years with the justification that patients must be protected from harming themselves. It is accepted that unfamiliarity with surroundings increases the likelihood of a fall that can result in injury. Also restrained are patients who have been known to wander or patients who are perceived as threats to other patients and staff. Restraints have also been used as part of behavior-modification programs.

Restraints can be physical, chemical, observant, or seclusive. Physical restraints include different types of patient tying, such as two-point or four-point systems, vests, equipment such as Adirondack chairs, which make standing up difficult, wheelchairs with lock-in bars. Chemical restraints are sometimes selected to modify the behavior of the patient. Observant restraint is the use of a one-on-one observer, who monitors the patient continuously and perhaps tries to modify the behavior. Seclusive restraint is the placement of a patient in a room without other human beings.

Nursing homes and medical wards of hospitals use restraints most frequently to prevent further harm from befalling the patients. For this problem, the restraint is usually physical in nature. Patients who have restraints placed on them are at risk for injuries that are directly related to the use of the restraint. There can be physical injuries such as skin trauma and psychological injuries such as anxiety at being immobilized. There can be long-term decrease in functional capacities as well as learned dependence on the restraints (Miles and Meyers 1994).

Many articles indicate that the physical restraints used in nursing homes are not particularly effective in reducing the number of falls suffered by residents (Evans and Strumpf 1989; Tinetti, Wen-Liang, Ginter 1992; Capezuti, Evans, et al. 1996). This evidence, combined with Medicare/Medicaid requirements for the presumption against physical restraints (Kapp 1992) has caused nursing homes to review their policies and create alternative care strategies (Schnelle, MacRae, et al. 1994; Werner, Koroknay, et al. 1996; Evans and Strumpf 1997).

In this specific case, the restraints being used were physical and observant. The patient apparently did not object to the physical restraint but did object to the observer, while the brother objected to the physical but not the observer. This may be indicative of the health capacities of each. The sister could not move out of bed without help. The presence of an uninvited human from whom she could not move away might be a psychological restraint, an invasion of her privacy. Her brother, who could move about, saw the vest as restrictive. The presence of others was not restrictive since he could move away.

Although the case reached a satisfactory conclusion, it is important that staff continue to monitor Ms. Eisen at night and to determine if, in fact, her brother's original hypothesis was correct or mistaken. That is, he speculated that the posey caused his sister to increase the danger to herself by inciting her to move about. This is an empirical question and one that the staff have a moral obligation to determine to the best of their ability.

REFERENCES

Elizabeth Capezuti, Lois Evans, Neville Strumpf, Greg Maislin, 1996. "Physical restraint use and falls in nursing home residents." *Journal of the American Geriatric Society* 44(6): 627–33.

Lois K. Evans, Neville E. Strumpf, S. Lynne Allen-Taylor, Elizabeth Capezuti, Greg Maislin, Barbara Jacobsen, 1997. "A clinical trial to reduce restraints in nursing homes." *Journal of the American Geriatric Society* 45(6): 675–81.

Lois K. Evans, Neville E. Strumpf, 1989. "Tying down the elderly." *Journal of the American Geriatric Society* 37(1):65–74.

Marshall B. Kapp, 1992. "Nursing home restraints and legal liability." *Journal of Legal Medicine* 13(1):1–32.

Steven H. Miles, Roberta Meyers, 1994. "Untying the elderly." *Clinics in Geriatric Medicine* 10(3): 513–25.

National Citizens' Coalition for Nursing Home Reform, 1996. *Individualized care approaches to reduce the use of chemical and physical restraints.* NCCNHR, Washington, DC.

John F. Schnelle, Priscilla G. Mac Rae, Sandra F. Simmons, Gwen Uman, Joseph G. Ouslander, Lori L. Rosenquist, Betty Chang, 1994. "Safety assessment for frail elderly: A comparison of restrained and unrestrained nursing home residents." *Journal of the American Geriatric Society* 42(6): 586–92.

Mary E. Tinetti, Liu Wen-Liang, Sandra R. Ginter, 1992. "Mechanical restraint use and fall-related injuries among residents of skilled nursing facilities." *Annals of Internal Medicine* 116(5):369–74.

Perla Werner, Vivian Koroknay, Judith Braun, Jiska Cohen-Mansfield, 1994. "Individualized care alternatives used in the process of removing physical restraints in the nursing home." *Journal of the American Geriatric Society* 42(3): 321–25.

Organizational and Institutional Ethics

Editors' Note: Fiscal and mission issues present themselves in many forms. As a result, we must vary our format in this section in order to present the situation as it was encountered in the institutions. Because the goal of the deliberation is usually institutional policy rather than resolution of a single case, the case descriptions are thinner.

Case Twenty-One:
A Memo About Our Mission

KEY TERMS: *Fiscal Scarcity, Organizational Ethics, Institutional Ethics, Mission Services, Indigent Care, Uninsured Patients*

NARRATIVE

Memorandum

To: Michael Bennett, M.A., M.Div.
Vice President for Mission Services

From: John O'Hara, M.D.
Director, Medical Staff

Philip Wong, Pharm.D.
Chairman, Formulary Committee

Subject: Nonpayment for prescription pharmaceuticals

We ask your insights regarding a pressing problem. This situation is acute. We have received administrative directives to recoup more of the delinquent charges owed to our respective departments. Can you advise us regarding the ramifications, for the mission and values of our hospital, of several courses of action under consideration?

We have a serious problem with nonpayment of emergency room (ER) bills. Many patients come to the ER for care instead of going to a physician's office. As you know, this is old news. Of note is the fact that not all of these are "self-pay" patients (i.e., uninsured persons from whom we can seldom collect charges). Some are Medicare patients, and some have other kinds of insurance. For instance, a patient might realize that it will take a long time to get in to see the family doctor, but they can come to the ER at a slow time and be seen immediately. That, in itself, is a resource allocation issue with ethical implications but one that we can't tackle very easily because of the Emergency Medical Treatment and Labor Act (EMTALA). And it would just plain make us and our staff uncomfortable to turn people away who presented for treatment.

The problem we'd like to address concerns prescription drugs for this same patient population. Often these patients will claim not to have the money to have their prescriptions filled, or they'll point out (e.g., at

2:00 A.M.) that all the other pharmacies are closed, and ask that the hospital pharmacy fill this script. They will then pay by saying "just put it on my bill." This is often a bill that either (a) will never be paid if they are uninsured or (b) will be paid at a greatly reduced rate by Medicare. (Medicare doesn't pay at all for outpatient medications.) Some of the Medicare patients seem to premeditate this situation. Cases are reported in which patients will come in late at night and say, "Well, I'm sick 'cause I don't have my medicines." The ER doctor will write prescriptions for several items that will then be tacked onto their bill. This is an institutionalized way of losing money in a manner that may not be a part of our mission. Is our mission being served in these cases in ways not obvious to us? Furthermore, we wish remedies that will not be in violation of our desire to serve the indigent. In our effort to curb abuses of the system, we do not wish to create problems for those with legitimate needs.

What should we do in these cases? The Pharmacy Department is losing a good deal of money this way. Some wish to create a policy that simply says "no filling outpatient prescriptions without payment." Obviously we don't want to go that far. We realize there are genuinely poor patients who need the help and charity for which our hospital is known. Some other ideas include (a) fill the prescription for several days of medication to assist the patient until he or she can access some other help for payment, (b) develop a database to help identify repeat users/abusers of the system, (c) give each ER physician a certain amount of "money" to use for prescription purposes, i.e., a limited amount of credit designed to motivate them to judge more judiciously, or (d) have the social worker called on each case. (As you might imagine, the physicians are none too happy about idea #c; the social workers are concerned about the potential additional workload created by #d).

Any ideas or help you can give us regarding what our hospital can do to both be more fiscally prudent and still serve those we seek to serve, will be appreciated.

Memorandum

To: John O'Hara, M.D.
          Director, Medical Staff

          Philip Wong, Pharm.D.
          Chairman, Formulary Committee

From: Michael Bennett, M.A., M.Div.
          Vice President for Mission Services

Subject: Nonpayment for prescription pharmaceuticals

Thank you for your memo requesting input from the Mission Service perspective on the problem of nonpayment of prescriptions given to ER patients. You are certainly raising an appropriate question, and I think some of your proposed solutions have merit from a mission-values point of view.

Certainly it is consistent with our mission to expect payment for the services we render. If that were not the case, our mission would end very quickly as we slipped into bankruptcy. Indeed, lack of profitability threatens our ability to maintain many of our most important community service programs. Of course, our mission does include a preferential option for the poor, and this preference has been manifested in various ways, one way being our provision of charitable care. This principle of the preferential option for the poor compels us to provide care for those who do not have the financial means to reimburse us, especially when they do not have other options.

As you are probably aware, unpaid bills or bad debt cannot be later reclassified or "booked" as charitable care, so it is important to us as an organization that our charitable care be identified as that from the beginning. This is becoming even more important as our not-for-profit status is being challenged by some municipalities and by our for-profit competitors.

Apart from the principles that guide our mission, there are also some practical considerations that I'm sure you have thought about. It makes little sense to expend several hundred dollars on an ER visit for a patient with no funds, and then not spend the extra fifty dollars to fill the prescription that will avoid having the patient return to the ER the next night with the same problem. This same practical consideration holds true for paying patients who might be temporarily short of cash but who need their prescriptions filled immediately.

My recommendations, based on your suggestions, are as follows:

1. The pharmacy should have a general rule that all outpatient prescriptions are "cash and carry" with the exceptions noted below.
2. For patients who temporarily do not have funds—e.g. they forgot their wallet or checkbook—a seventy-two-hour supply will be dispensed, and the patient can return and pick up the remainder of the prescription when they have cash.
3. For patients who cannot pay because of financial hardship, a seventy-two-hour supply will be dispensed by the pharmacy. The patient will also be given a referral card to call or see the ER social worker either immediately (if it's during business hours) or the next business day. The seventy-two-hour supply will ensure an adequate amount of medication to cover even a

long holiday weekend. The social worker will assess the patient's financial situation, investigate other funding sources,
e.g., Title XIX, Veterans Relief, the County Pharmacy etc. For
those patients with true financial hardship and no alternative
methods of payment, the remainder of the prescription will be
filled and charged to the charity fund. The social worker will
maintain a database of persons who are assisted in such a fashion to track users of the system and avoid having to repeat this
procedure each time such a patient requires a prescription.
"Abusers" of the system could be handled on a case-by-case
basis.

I understand from discussions with medical and pharmacy staff
that the above recommendations are not without pitfalls. A specific
worry involves antibiotics. There is a concern that patients will take
seventy-two hours worth of their antibiotic, begin to feel better, and
then neglect to get the remainder filled. In response to this problem,
pharmacy staff must maintain a commitment to counseling the patients
on the importance of taking the prescribed antibiotic for the full course
of therapy. We will, therefore, be giving people the information they
need to make an informed decision and empower them to take responsibility for their own actions. An exception will be made for antibiotic
suspensions for children. Since these are usually dispensed in premeas-
ured ten-day supplies, and since children should not be held responsible for an irresponsible choice by their parents, the full ten-day supply of antibiotics will be dispensed. But the social service referral will
still be initiated.

My hope is that the above steps will significantly reduce the amount
of prescription drugs that are "put on the bill" with little chance of being
paid for or reimbursed by a third-party payer while insuring that we are
not turning away those who truly need our charitable care.

COMMENTARY

This kind of case is an antidote to the cynicism that pervades many current discussions of health-care reform and cost cutting. Such discussions often portray all reform and reorganization as brutal to patient
care and quality delivery of services, and then either decry this situation or justify it as necessary to save the nation from financial ruin. As
is evident in this current case, the reality is often quite different.

Administrators must grapple with ways to reduce costs or to recoup payment for services rendered. As noted by the vice president for
mission services, there is nothing inherently "dirty" about these goals

of sound fiscal management. In fact, achieving these goals often enables the institution to better serve those most in need and is also simply required by the moral obligation not to waste resources (Ubel and Arnold 1995). But the specific means to the goals must be examined one by one to be sure that the mission and values of the institution are not compromised by the details of a proposal. As a result, this vice president was willing to support certain proposals while challenging application of these same initiatives to highly vulnerable populations (e.g., children).

As demonstrated by the concern that some patients will not complete their course of antibiotics, it is difficult to craft solutions that carry no risk of raising new problems. But when all things were considered, the hospital simply had to ask some patients to share more responsibility for the administration of their treatment as a cost-containment measure. This kind of policy obviously will need to be monitored and reviewed at intervals to ascertain its effects. A commitment to vigilant oversight and the implementation of effective feedback mechanisms are characteristic of caring professionals (Woodstock Theological Center 1995, 32) and caring institutions (Scott, Aiken, et al. 1995).

REFERENCES

Robert A. Scott, Linda H. Aiken, David Mechanic, Julius Moravcsik, 1995. "Organizational aspects of caring." *Milbank Memorial Fund Quarterly* 73(1): 77–95.

Peter A. Ubel, Robert M. Arnold, 1995. "The unbearable rightness of bedside rationing." *Archives of Internal Medicine* 155:1837–42.

Woodstock Theological Center, 1995. *Ethical considerations in the business aspects of health care*, Washington, DC: Georgetown University Press.

FOR FURTHER READING

Stanley Joel Reiser, 1994. "The ethical life of health care organizations," *Hastings Center Report* 24(6):28–35.

Case Twenty-Two:
Who Pays? Hospital Coping Strategies in a Managed Care Environment[1]

KEY TERMS: *Fiscal Scarcity, Organizational Ethics, Institutional Ethics, Patient Autonomy*

Consider the following scenarios:

1. A patient is medically ready for discharge, but has no support at home until the next day. Consequently, the physician orders an additional hospital day before discharge, for which the payer refuses to pay the hospital because it is medically unnecessary.

2. A postsurgical patient needed blood prior to discharge. Although the blood was readily available and discharge could have occurred soon after administration, the patient insisted on donor-directed blood, which would result in prolonging the hospital stay by three days. After considerable discussion, the patient was offered the choice of accepting the available blood, paying for the additional stay, or being discharged "against medical advice" (AMA) and returning for donor-directed blood, when available, as an outpatient. This last option obviously involved some additional risk to the patient. Nevertheless, the patient chose this riskier course, which was accomplished without incident.

THE LANGUAGE AND ISSUES OF THE CASE

Cases of this kind bring a variety of terms and issues to the fore. Clearly, at issue is what patients are entitled to expect from the health-care system. Medical ethics often speaks about patient autonomy, but this is usually conceived negatively in terms of being free from unwanted treatment. Here, we must ask whether respecting patient autonomy

---

1. This case and the accompanying commentary first appeared as Andrew Thurman, 1995. "Managed care for healthcare providers." *Community ethics: The newsletter of the consortium ethics program* 3(1): 9–10.

brings certain entitlements with it. How far may they direct the choice of treatments? Are certain social needs or idiosyncratic preferences to be included under the heading of health care?

COMMENTARY

Many assert that managed care, with its inherent inducement to withhold services, is unethical. If health care is considered a commodity, then such an assertion is clearly inaccurate. But if a certain level of basic health care is (or should be) a right, as most health-care providers and bioethicists seem to believe, then any reimbursement system which causes either the underutilization or overutilization of resources is unethical. A good managed care plan is meant to adjust the level of care so that neither extreme occurs. Managed care is a reality and providers must learn to deal with its reimbursement policies in a way that helps to facilitate the right amount of care. This will involve bedside calculations by the physician and the hospital administration (Ubel and Arnold 1995; Ubel and Goold 1997).

The scenarios above occurred in a market in which managed care mainly takes the form of fee-for-service reimbursement with a managed care overlay. That is, physicians and hospitals each receive reimbursement for the specific services they render. But the insurer only reimburses "medically necessary" services as defined by guidelines they have developed in concert with the hospital and its medical staff (a system known as "clinical pathways"). When the physician or hospital attempts to bill for services that are beyond those noted in the guidelines, the insurer will not pay unless an explanation can be provided that shows the "medical necessity" of the additional services. At one time, such social as well as medical goals could easily be served by the medical system. But shrinking resources make this difficult, and if such goals are to be met by the health-care system, the question of "who pays?" cannot be avoided.

As managed care spreads, providers will find innovative alternatives, such as home care, to resolve the first kind of scenario. The patient's need for help at home is a kind of health-care need, but is no longer one that is seen as requiring the resources available within a hospital (Shortell, Gillies, and Devers 1995; Stoeckle 1995). But until that happens, the hospital probably should not be forced to "eat" this loss—it should be the responsibility of the patient or the ordering physician. But if the payer refuses to reimburse the hospital for a day's stay that the physician and the hospital believe is medically necessary, the hospital should pursue all legal remedies against the payer. Because the physician and the hospital see no way to keep this patient physically safe without keeping her for this extra day, it is probably ethically acceptable to see the patient's need as medical in nature and to bill for it. Even though such a strategy is not effective on a case-by-case basis, experience has shown that this strategy can alter the behavior of the payer over the long term.

Managed care payers may be found legally liable when they deny authorization for medically necessary care. Providers, however, will always have liability risk when they choose not to provide services because payment for those services has been denied. The proper course for providers, when they believe services are medically necessary, is to provide those services and then aggressively pursue the payer for payment.

In the second case, the patient has an idiosyncratic preference for treatment that is not considered to be necessary according to standard care. Extra days of hospital stay to accomplish such marginal benefit will not be reimbursed by the insurer. The hospital has a duty of beneficence to the patient, but it has no obligation to use its scarce charity care resources to meet patients' unusual preferences. It would seem more just for the institution to channel its resources to the truly indigent in need of basic care. As a result, it had to ask this patient to assume the costs of the additional hospitalization or to assume the risks brought on by discharge. In this case, the patient chose to assume the risk. Nevertheless, it is difficult to know a priori if the hospital would have faced some risk of liability should this patient have been injured during the three days prior to transfusion.

In sum, the challenge of managed care to providers is to determine, and aggressively enforce, who should bear the cost of services provided. If the services are medically necessary, the payer should pay. If the services are not medically necessary, then the patient or the responsible provider (usually the ordering physician) should bear the cost.

REFERENCES

Stephen M. Shortell, Robin R. Gillies, and Kelly J. Devers, 1995. "Reinventing the american hospital." *The Milbank Memorial Fund Quarterly* 73(2): 131–60.

John D. Stoeckle, 1995. "The citadel cannot hold: Technologies go outside the hospital, patients and doctors too." *Milbank Memorial Fund Quarterly* 73(1): 3–17.

Peter A. Ubel, Robert M. Arnold, 1995. "The unbearable rightness of bedside rationing." *Archives of Internal Medicine* 155:1837–42.

Peter A. Ubel, Susan Goold, 1997. "Bedside rationing: Clear cases and tough calls." *Annals of Internal Medicine* 126(1): 74–80.

FOR FURTHER READING

Stanley Joel Reiser, 1994. "The ethical life of health care organizations." *Hastings Center Report* 24(6):28–35.

Woodstock Theological Center, 1995. *Ethical considerations in the business aspects of health care*. Washington, DC: Georgetown University Press.

Case Twenty-Three:
Who's in Charge? Managed Care
and the Ethics Consultant

KEY TERMS: *Informed Consent, Surrogate Decision Making, Managed Care, Organizational Ethics, Institutional Ethics, Ethics Consultation, Deception, Truth Telling*

NARRATIVE

Mr. S, a 52-year-old male, was admitted three weeks ago. He had a stroke due to heart failure. He was initially treated aggressively and evaluated for a heart transplant. Although he began to breathe better and was taken off the mechanical ventilator, his mental functioning was extremely poor and did not improve. In fact, it continued to deteriorate to the point where the patient did not have any conscious awareness, although he occasionally opened his eyes. However, his eye movements and the noises he made were not discernibly purposeful.

The attending physician continually discussed the situation with the patient's family. The patient's wife, Mary, was at the bedside throughout most of the stay and an adult son visited every couple of days. After two weeks, the patient was made "all but CPR." In other words, he would get all aggressive care, but if his heart stopped, the medical team would not perform resuscitation. After three weeks, the family agreed that the patient should just be "kept comfortable." There were frequent conversations between physician and family to determine exactly what "being kept comfortable" would mean since the patient still had such things as a tube for nutrition and hydration, i.e., a nasogastric tube.

The hospital social worker was concerned. She realized that this patient's length of stay was becoming so long that the insurance company might later review the case and deny reimbursement for some of the patient's time in the hospital. If so, the family would be surprised to be getting a bill in the mail, since no one had told them their coverage was running out. The social worker continued to try to persuade the family that they should move the patient to a hospice. (This would resolve the course of treatment and the financial concerns since the patient's insurance covered a period of hospice care.) But she did not feel she should be the one discussing the finances of the case with the family during this

134

sensitive time. As a result, she called the ethics consultant and told him that he was needed because "the family was conflicted."

The ethics consultant discussed these end-of-life decisions with the family and then called the attending physician. The consultant thought that the family members were progressing nicely in their decision-making process. The attending physician seemed annoyed that the ethics consultant had been called and wondered aloud what the reason for the consult was. The ethics consultant shared some of this confusion as to his mission in the case. Only two days later did the social worker explain the financial difficulty to the consultant. At that time, the family still had not agreed to placement but wished Mr. S to be allowed to die in the hospital with comfort measures being administered.

The social worker was upset by the family's decision because Mr. S might take more hospital days to die than his insurance allowed. The ethics consultant asked the social worker how she knew about the financial issues involved. She explained that a case manager, who is a hospital employee familiar with the reimbursement guidelines of the insurer, monitored the case and reported to the attending physician but did not make any chart notes, since this was a kind of quality assurance activity. This case manager also makes treatment suggestions to the attending physician and notifies the attending about deviations from the clinical pathway. As a result, the evaluation of the reimbursement situation took place in a manner hidden from the ethics consultant and most members of the health-care team. The consultant was not quite sure what to do at this point.

THE LANGUAGE AND ISSUES OF THE CASE

The language of this case is contestable. One can view it as an issue of informed consent. That is, what information do surrogates need in order to make a fully informed decision? More specifically, we might ask the following questions.

1. Should financial matters, such as insurance reimbursement be discussed during decisions to forgo life-sustaining treatment? What standards of decision making should guide the patient's or family's choices in balancing the medical, social, and financial factors? How should health-care providers counsel families regarding the role of financial considerations in making life-and-death decisions?
2. Who, if anyone, is responsible for discussing financial matters with patients and families during hospital stays? Should this be the attending physician or does that undermine the doctor-

patient-family relationship? Should the case manager have to
issue regular reports to the family? Is it legitimate for this level
of surveillance (i.e., the case manager) to be hidden from the
family's and the ethics consultant's view? Is it legitimate to see
these managers as quality assurance persons and therefore
claim they are not participants in the decision-making process?
3.   Should ethics consultants be called upon to raise this kind of
issue with a patient's family? What is the role of this particular
ethics consultant in this case?

PERSPECTIVES AND KEY POINTS OF VIEW

The Attending Physician: He did not see a problem and was
slightly annoyed at all the "chatter" surrounding the case. He was not
interested in the ethics consultation. This was understandable given
that the real reason for the consult was not available to the consultant.
The attending physician believed that he was handling the discussions
with the family well and that issues of reimbursement should not play
a part in these talks. He generally did not think that the cost of several
unreimbursed hospital days should be a factor in end-of-life decision
making.

The Case Manager: The case manager saw the attending physician as being a little too passive in guiding the decision to forgo treatment and in not bringing the placement issue to a swifter conclusion.
Nevertheless, the hospital would still clearly be reimbursed for all care
up to that point. So, the situation had not been urgent.

The case manager had offered to help facilitate the family's decision-
making process but the attending declined this intervention. However, if
matters were not resolved soon, the case manager would have to notify
his supervisor, a faculty physician called the "line manager." Under the
system in this facility, the line manager is empowered to be quite aggressive and can even write discharge orders.

The Patient's Wife (Mary) and Son: They were grief-stricken
about the sudden loss of Mr. S. Nevertheless, they gradually came to
accept that he would not get better. They were quite clear that if Mr. S
was not going to get better, he would not want to be kept alive "on machines." They would like him to be made comfortable and were confused by the repeated discussions of moving him to a hospice or some
other facility. They had no idea why anyone would want to move a
dying man when he only had a few days left. The hospital staff, espe-

cially the social worker, seemed cold, pushy, and annoying to them. But they liked the ethics consultant and felt good about talking through their decisions with him. However, he didn't seem to have anything to do with the question of transfer.

The Ethics Consultant: The ethics consultant was in the dark for most of the consultation. He responded as he normally would to a case that was described as the family not being able to come to a firm decision about treatment. He had several discussions with the patient's family, and it was clear that they knew, in general terms, what the patient would want. The consultant discussed specific issues such as the possible removal of the feeding tube. He helped them to understand that such a choice was not unusual in similar cases and would be consistent with the treatment goals. He gave them opportunities to express their grief. However, once the consultant learned that he was actually involved in a fiscal matter, he was not sure how to proceed. This did not seem to be the kind of information that ethics consultants should be directly conveying to families. He was also very concerned to learn that there was a layer of decision making (i.e., the case manager) that did not make entries in the patient's medical record. This seemed contrary to the standard principles of a team approach to health care.

The Social Worker: The social worker did not want to discuss financial matters with the family. She did not believe that to be her place unless the attending physician delegated it to her. But she also did not want the family to receive a surprise invoice in the mail in the future for unreimbursed hospital days. She thought that everything would be fine if the family would just hurry up and make some decisions. So, she called the ethics consultant in order to speed the process.

WHAT ACTUALLY HAPPENED

The ethics consultant called the chair of the ethics committee (EC) and asked if the consultant's role was defined regarding financial matters. The chair suggested that the consultant could easily raise this issue among all the caregivers involved but that it was best if the consultant was not the one to inform the family regarding issues of insurance coverage. However, the consultant continued to be superfluous since his discussions with the attending physician were, like those of the social worker, of the "hurry up" variety. That is, he tried to persuade the attending physician that it was important to raise these issues with the family. But this effort was to no avail.

The attending continued to speak with the family each day. The patient's wife eventually agreed to move her husband to a hospice facility. However, this was on a Friday, and the transfer could not be arranged until the following week. Mr. S died on Sunday night. Although it could not be stated with certainty at the time, it was possible that the insurance company might retroactively deny coverage for as many as five days.

COMMENTARY

The simplest issues are often the most profound. We have only recently become a bit more comfortable with talking about death. And just when we were starting to make some progress, we must figure out how to talk about death and money. There is no easy way to do this but we can say several things about this case:

1. Patients or their surrogate decision makers have a right to all material information in helping to form a treatment plan. Thus, they clearly need to be informed about the financial impact of their treatment choices.
2. The idea of a "quality assurance" person who monitors the utilization of services and the patient's length of stay is morally neutral in itself. However, when this person has an impact on the formulation of the treatment plan or can even issue treatment directives (as in the case of the line manager), that person has an obligation to be accessible to the patient and family and to record his or her observations in the medical record. At that point, this person is no longer acting in only a quality assurance capacity.
3. Whether ethics consultants can give patients and their families information independent of that provided by the treatment team is controversial. For instance, ethics consultants are sometimes the first person to say the word "death" to a family. Some claim that this is diagnostic information and properly the province of the attending physician. Whatever one thinks of that long-running issue, one thing is clear: The ethics consultant should certainly not be the person delegated to breaking financial bad news to a family. This role clearly belongs to someone else, and it is the job of each institution to define precisely who that is and to be sure that it is usually done reasonably well.
4. Although there is no particular person who intrinsically should be the one to discuss finances with the patient and/or family, we should realize that institutionalizing and routinizing such a

role presents a great opportunity. Too often prognostic statements have remained vague. For instance, in a case like that of Mr. S, a physician will initially state to the family that "It's too early to tell" whether he will get better. This is true enough. But it leaves the family wondering when they will know more. The case manager has guidelines in front of him or her that are far more precise. What family wouldn't rather be told that "We anticipate about five days of the initial treatment and observation. We hope he will then be responding to the experimental therapy. If he isn't showing some improvement by then, we'll know that he is unlikely to benefit from aggressive treatment. We will know then a lot more about his chances of recovery, and we'll have to consider other options." Despite the fact that this mixes hope and potential failure in the initial message, it is probably the kind of frank discussion a family would prefer. The anger in the present case seems to have resulted from the withholding of information—not from giving bad news.

5. In bringing cases such as this one to an ethics committee for retrospective review, ethics consultants are able to facilitate opportunities to assess managed care policies in action. As hospitals make the transition from fee-for-service to managed care, there is a tremendous opportunity for health-care professionals to continually reassess the effects of policies and to advocate specific changes to facilitate better patient care.

In closing, it is interesting to note the language of the caregivers in characterizing the case. The social worker is the person who most wished to give full disclosure of the financial situation to the family. Nevertheless, when she called the ethics consultant, she characterized the issue as something that was wrong with the patient's family, i.e., they were "conflicted." It is a good idea for an ethics consultant always to take the stated "reason" for the consult with a grain of salt. Ethics consultation often involves reconstructing the narrative of the case to make the salient ethical issues clear. This particular case highlights how perennial issues of medical ethics such as truth telling, deception, and communication reemerge within the managed care context.

FOR FURTHER READING

Paul S. Appelbaum, 1993. "Must we forgo informed consent to control health care costs? A response to Mark A. Hall." *Milbank Memorial Fund Quarterly* 71(4):669–77.

Ruth R. Faden, 1997. "Managed care and informed consent." *Kennedy Institute of Ethics Journal* 7(4):377–79.

Mark A. Hall, 1993. "Informed consent to rationing decisions." *Milbank Memorial Fund Quarterly* 71(4):645–67. (See also 1994, "Disclosing rationing decisions: A reply to Paul S. Appelbaum," *Milbank Quarterly*, 72(2):211–15.)

David Mechanic, 1994. "Trust and informed consent to rationing." *Milbank Memorial Fund Quarterly* 72(2):217–23.

Frances H. Miller, 1992. "Denial of health care and informed consent in English and American law." *American Journal of Law and Medicine*, 18(1&2):37–71.

SECTION SIX

Rehabilitation Ethics

Case Twenty-Four:
This Is Consent to Therapy?

KEY TERMS: *Rehabilitation Ethics, Informed Consent, Process Models of Informed Consent, Noncompliance*

NARRATIVE

Mr. X was a 70-year-old man with a history of severe back pain for almost a decade. Mr. X was formerly a proud steel worker. This pain contributed to his decision to take an early retirement buyout from a local company about ten years ago. The pain increased in recent months and radiated downward from the lower back into his legs.

Since retirement, Mr. X has gained a good deal of weight, although two attempts to control it resulted in significant weight losses. He denied that his weight was linked to his back pain but his medical records made it seem likely that it was. Mr. X's lifestyle included occasional alcohol consumption, and he smoked a pack of cigarettes each day. His medical history was also significant for rheumatoid arthritis and chronic obstructive pulmonary disease (COPD).

Mr. X's mood was quite variable. It was observed that when he went to his various therapies (e.g., physical therapy, occupational therapy), he participated well and seemed to make some progress. Unfortunately, every morning Mr. X refused therapy, stating that it was "[expletives deleted] awful that he has to be taken care of like a little baby," or that his pain was too much that day. When asked by the nursing staff why he was not going to therapy, he sometimes said, "What's the use?"

Mr. X had a 33-year-old son, Skip, who was a banker. Skip was married and had two children. He said that his father was always a fighter, and he believed his father could be so again. If Mr. X could get to the point where he could take care of most of his daily living functions ("If he just doesn't stay in bed all day"), Skip and his wife would like Mr. X to live with them. If not, Mr. X would have to find some sort of a structured living situation.

THE LANGUAGE AND ISSUES OF THE CASE

This case is likely to be discussed in terms of the language of informed consent. In particular, we will have to determine whether the therapists are merely persuading Mr. X to attend therapy or are coercing him. This will require that we decide which of Mr. X's statements express his autonomy, those he makes in the morning or those he states after he is engaged in therapy. Let us list the issues succinctly.

1. Is it okay for the therapists to be somewhat forceful in getting Mr. X. to therapy? Is Mr. X competent to make these choices?
2. Is it okay to enlist the help of others such as family in persuading Mr. X.? To what extent? When does consent to therapy actually occur—when he was admitted and signed a general consent to treatment form? At a weekly review of his treatment plan? Each morning?
3. Would an ethics consultant's recommendation change if (a) Mr. X had a less active history, e.g., was a sedentary homemaker his entire life? (b) Mr. X had an unsupportive family? (c) Mr. X had a less hopeful prognosis, e.g., he was an oncology rehabilitation patient with a bleak five-year survival probability?

PERSPECTIVES AND KEY POINTS OF VIEW

The Treatment Team: There are many persons involved in Mr. X's care, plus a variety of sentiments. Although opinions are not uniform across specialties, some generalizations can be made on the basis of profession.

In general, the physical and occupational therapists emphasize that Mr. X generally responds positively to therapy once he is engaged in it. So they believe that being aggressive in getting Mr. X to therapy is warranted. They believe therapy is what Mr. X really wants and that "you shouldn't take his morning crankiness too seriously."

Meanwhile, the nursing staff takes what Mr. X says very seriously. They believe that the therapists often fail to respect a competent adult's wishes and violate his rights as a patient. They think he needs more empathy and care and a little less therapy.

The social worker is torn between these two trains of thought. On the one hand, her role as the patient's advocate leads her to agree with the nurses. On the other, she realizes that Mr. X will not meet the insurance criteria to remain a rehabilitation patient unless he fulfills the minimal daily therapy requirements. Although it is his right to be transferred to a less demanding environment such as a nursing home, the social worker believes that such an outcome would "be a shame," because otherwise Mr. X could live with his son and might even be capable of more independence.

Skip (patient's son): He loves his father and would like to help him. However, Skip feels strongly that he must be realistic and require that his father be able to take basic care of himself before he (Skip) can agree to have him live with his family. Skip, like his father, is a realist and will not sacrifice his family to around-the-clock caregiving.

Mr. X: We have little insight into the workings of Mr. X's mind other than what we have already heard. Like many patients, he seems ambivalent. When he has been productive at therapy, he seems to place a normal value on routine living. When he must again begin his "daily grind," he evidences a more negative evaluation of his situation.

POSSIBLE ALTERNATIVE ENDINGS

The major question is whether Mr. X is willing to cooperate with at least the minimal therapy regimen necessary for him to obtain benefits from his stay and to continue to qualify as a rehabilitation candidate. The staff must find a way of determining whether Mr. X ultimately believes continued therapy is in his best interest. Furthermore, if Mr. X wishes to continue in therapy, it will be helpful to learn if there are ways to make his therapy regimen more palatable to him.

WHAT ACTUALLY HAPPENED

Discussion of the situation with Mr. X and selected members of his treatment team determined the following:

1. Mr. X finds his occasional loss of bowel control during therapy to be so humiliating that he wishes to scrap the entire regimen and give up. This problem is what he meant by needing to "be taken care of like a little baby."
2. Mr. X generally likes physical and occupational therapy. However, there are one or two range-of-movement exercises that he finds especially difficult and painful and not necessary to his life.

The treatment team worked with Mr. X. to devise ways to keep his therapy more secluded from the observation of other patients during times when he was especially vulnerable to loss of bowel control. The therapists also discussed with him alternative exercises that they would try with him that might meet the same goals as the ones that he so disliked. He agreed to try the new routine for one week, and then the therapists would again discuss his progress with him. Mr. X agreed that for that trial week, the therapist could "push" him hard to complete the new routine.

COMMENTARY

Informed consent is often best conceived as a process. This is especially true in rehabilitation (Caplan, Callahan, and Haas 1987). The treatment team correctly noted that Mr. X's initial agreement to work toward his rehabilitation goals was a part of the informed consent process and that this initial agreement was relevant to his daily refusals. Of course, they needed to be reminded that the process is ongoing and that Mr. X's current sentiments must also be considered.

Informed consent always requires a blending of overall treatment goals and particular treatments or therapies (Haas 1993). In this case, the patient sometimes made statements about overall goals (e.g., "What's the use?"). But, the treatment team did well to question the motivations for these statements and to discuss with Mr. X the particular problems he was having in therapy. Compromises were reached on certain therapies, and the therapists had a clear way to proceed for the following week. Once things were examined in this perspective, Mr. X's seeming "noncompliance" vanished (Scofield 1995).

As is so often the case, the major problem the patient was having was hidden from the treatment team. In rehabilitation care, issues of patient privacy and dignity often come to the fore.

Rehabilitation professionals sometimes stress that the camaraderie of the therapy room and the social aspects of rehabilitation care can help a patient, but it is also important to be aware when such a public environment might also be compromising a particular patient's care. Had Mr. X's sentiments in this regard remained hidden, they would have continued to undermine his entire plan of care and his opportunity to benefit from the available therapy.

REFERENCES

Arthur L. Caplan, Daniel Callahan, Janet Haas, 1987. "Ethical and policy issues in rehabilitation medicine." *Hastings Center Report*, Special Supplement, 17:S1–S19.

Janet Haas, 1993. "Ethical considerations of goal setting for patient care in rehabilitation medicine." *American Journal of Physical Medicine and Rehabilitation* 72(4):228–32.

Giles R. Scofield, 1995. "The problem of (non-)compliance: Is it patients or patience?" *HEC Forum* 7(2–3):150–65.

FOR FURTHER READING

Karen Grandstand Gervais, Dorothy E. Vawter, and Emily Spilseth, 1995. "Readings in rehabilitation ethics." *HEC Forum* 7(2):183–97.

Ruth B. Purtilo, 1984. "Applying the principles of informed consent to patient care: Legal and ethical considerations for physical therapy." *Physical Therapy* 64:934–37.

Ruth B. Purtilo, 1988. "Ethical issues in teamwork: The context of rehabilitation." *Archives of Physical Medicine and Rehabilitation* 69(5):318–22.

Case Twenty-Five:
Who's the Patient?[1]

KEY TERMS: *Rehabilitation Ethics, Surrogate Decision Making for Minors, Best Interests Standard, Support Groups, Family in Medical Decision Making*

NARRATIVE

JP was a four-year-old boy with spastic quadriplegia secondary to cerebral palsy (CP). He was also delayed intellectually and functioned at an 18-month-old level. When JP was six months old, his developmental pediatrician referred him to a pediatric program at St. Catherine's Rehabilitation Hospital for a comprehensive program of physical, occupational, speech, and hydro therapy. JP was the fourth of four children. His sisters were seven, nine, and 11 years of age. There were no other significant medical issues or history in the family.

Over the course of the past three-and-one-half years, JP and his parents had become quite interactive with the pediatric staff of the rehabilitation hospital. His mother and father took turns bringing him to therapy; they never brought him together. Once, JP's mother confided to the social worker that she thought their marriage was "on the rocks." She and her husband had wanted a son desperately, and when they found out about JP's developmental difficulties, things were never the same. Mrs. P felt she had failed as a wife and saw her main role as helping JP to be as normal as possible. She would do whatever she felt was necessary to achieve this end. She became active in local and state CP advocacy organizations, attended CP support groups, and was also quite active in her local school system. Mr. P was more passive; he watched therapy and took instructions home but didn't interact with JP any more than was necessary. Mr. P stated he loves his family, but it was hard for him to see his boy as a "helpless cripple."

From a therapeutic standpoint, JP's parents were able to understand and carry out a stretching/range-of-motion program and did an excellent job of maintaining this program. JP was able to stand with

---

1. This case, with a different commentary, originally appeared as Sarah Schlieper, 1996. "Who's the patient? A case study and commentary." *Community Ethics: The Newsletter of the Consortium Ethics Program* 3(3):4–5.

moderate support and had been doing so for about six months. He was able to take a step or two in the pool with assistance, which has become a "crowning achievement" for Mrs. P. The speech therapist had been working with JP on swallowing. JP had a gastric tube for three years and only recently had been able to attempt therapeutic feeds of pureed foods. Mrs. P stated she had given JP solid food on occasion, and he especially liked McDonald's french fries. She noticed that JP coughed sometimes when he tried them. However, she stated that tasting french fries and swimming are the only pleasures he had, and she doesn't feel the speech therapist should be taking one of these pleasures away from him. JP had one episode of aspiration pneumonia.

The treatment team had met by themselves and also with the physiatrist who was the attending physician for the pediatric program. In their professional opinion, JP would probably never ambulate, and if he got to the point where he could take a step or two on dry land, it would probably be with much assistance and not functional or safe. They met with Mrs. P to tell her their opinion.

Mrs. P's response was to state that there were several mothers in her CP organizations whose doctors said the same thing about their kids. Mrs. P added that as long as she never gives up hope, he would walk. JP was to begin kindergarten in two months, where he would receive educationally based physical therapy, occupational therapy, and speech therapy. The therapy team felt JP should be discharged from the pediatric program, except for speech therapy to monitor the swallowing situation (a medical issue) when he started kindergarten. The team thought his other therapeutic needs would be met by his individual educational program in kindergarten. When the physiatrist discussed termination with Mrs. P, she got quite angry and threatened to sue.

Mrs. P stated that JP's developmental pediatrician thought this recommendation was "insane" and would write orders for JP to continue all therapies, especially the pool. Mrs. P said that she sees progress constantly and that what the therapists were doing helped him. She also believed that speech therapy is the least of his needs and that he was ready to eat everything the family ate except tough meat. The therapy team discussed this informally over lunch, and most of them thought that JP's mother was overly involved with him and in denial. The therapists felt compromised at the idea of being forced to continue therapy even though they saw limited functional gains.

THE LANGUAGE AND ISSUES OF THE CASE

The language of the case will, to some degree, follow whichever issue one identifies as paramount. On the one hand, there is the simple issue regarding informed consent. Although we usually focus on consent, the information part can be at issue. The treatment team believes JP has reached a "plateau" and will not progress much. But plateaus in rehabilitation can be somewhat subjective, and we do not know if they have adequately prepared Mrs. P to see the plateau as impending and are accurately assessing the situation (e.g., should the information Mrs. P obtains at a support group be so easily dismissed?).

However, we can also choose to focus on the swallowing issue that Mrs. P believes is a nonissue. JP has had a bout of aspiration pneumonia probably attributable to these feedings. Is this evidence that Mrs. P is not able to care for her child properly or is engaged in some form of child abuse? This raises additional questions.

1. What was the treatment contract? What did the professionals and Mrs. P agree to when they began treatment? In other words, what information was given and when did consent occur? Has the process of informed consent continued? Have the treatment goals been revisited at appropriate intervals?
2. Is Mrs. P's ability to serve as a surrogate decision maker in question?
3. Are there child abuse/protection issues related to feeding JP? Should the staff of the rehabilitation hospital report this case to the local Children and Youth Services agency?
4. Do ethical conflicts exist among the professionals? That is, is there a conflict between the developmental pediatrician and the hospital staff that needs to be mediated?

PERSPECTIVES AND KEY POINTS OF VIEW

Mrs. P: Mrs. P is very adamant about the fact that JP still needs therapy as a medical treatment and that termination would do him and the family harm. She has educated herself through various special organizations and has been cooperative and compliant with all treatment and educational efforts until this point, except for the recent feeding issues. When asked about the feeding concerns, Mrs. P states that the speech therapist is "a nice girl, but she doesn't know what she's talking about." Mrs. P says that JP doesn't cough that much when he eats at McDonald's, and that she knows CPR and the Heimlich maneuver if he does start to choke. Mrs. P states she is willing to do whatever it takes to see JP continue in therapy, even if it means obtaining a lawyer. She says that the developmental pediatrician supports her point of view and feels JP needs to continue therapy.

Mr. P: He states that all medical and therapy decisions are Mrs. P's and that he doesn't have much to say when it comes to JP.

The Physiatrist: He believes that from a medical standpoint, JP's prognosis for functional walking is poor, yet he may be able to have a viable means of locomotion using a motorized wheelchair. He tried to approach this issue with Mrs. P, who refused to consider using a wheel-chair as a treatment goal. The physiatrist believes that therapy at this point is maintenance, yet acknowledges that "maintenance" is a gray area at best and that "in the old days" they would have kept JP in ther-apy even at the maintenance level. The physiatrist is reluctant to dis-agree with the developmental pediatrician but states that therapy and mobility in his opinion have plateaued, and that unless Mrs. P was to consider the use of a motorized chair in the future, and JP developed the skills needed to use the chair, physical therapy, occupational ther-apy, and hydro therapy should end. The physiatrist thinks that the only pertinent remaining medical issue is the feeding issue, which could be addressed by speech therapy. However, he said that Mrs. P is going to do what she wants regardless of medical recommendations.

The Therapists: They voice several concerns. They are concerned about Mrs. P, because they have gotten to known her well over the past few years and have seen her exhaust herself on JP's behalf. The physical therapist (PT) and occupational therapist (OT) agree that they have done all they can in terms of educating Mr. and Mrs. P in regard to JP's ongoing care. They believe that he has plateaued, and at this point the focus needs to shift toward the school and his "real life successes." The therapists emphasize they are not recommending stopping all therapy but that therapy does need to shift to the educational setting where JP's OT and PT needs will be met.

The speech therapist is concerned that Mrs. P is in denial about the feeding concerns and that JP is at risk for aspiration and choking. The speech therapist voices frustration with Mrs. P and has taken numer-ous approaches to try to discuss these issues with her. The speech ther-apist agrees that they are polarized and getting nowhere. She believes there will be progress in JP's ability to swallow safely, but it will take some time.

The Social Worker: She is concerned about the emotional status of the family and Mrs. P. The social worker thinks that marriage and family intervention around JP and the parents' experience of having a handicapped son would be beneficial to them emotionally. Improving their mental and emotional status might also help them to adhere to the new treatment regimen. However, there are no insurance funds available for this intervention, and the local Mental Health Department has a nine-month waiting list. In any event, Mrs. P is reluctant to try the Mental Health Department because of what she's heard in her advocacy groups. Mr. P states he is willing to try, but he is concerned that Mrs. P wouldn't get involved. The social worker is also concerned about the frustration of the team and their polarized position with Mrs. P. Because of the future risk of JP aspirating (Mrs. P's feeding attempts), the social worker wonders whether there is a child abuse issue here or the potential for one.

WHAT ACTUALLY HAPPENED

This team met again with Mr. and Mrs. P to review the recommendations and solicit their feedback. The team's agenda focused on concern around the feeding issue, the need to terminate physical therapy, occupational therapy, and hydro therapy, and the switch to an educational focus. Mrs. P seemed to focus on concerns that she and JP were being abandoned and being told there was no hope. The team was able to reframe some of these concerns so that the "graduation" from the program was seen as a move forward, not backward. The team and the parents were able to contract for periodic reevaluations of JP's rehabilitation status, with the understanding that when JP is able and ready to benefit from more intervention he would be considered for an outpatient program.

The physiatrist asked for and received permission to reinforce this plan with the pediatrician. The team also evaluated norm setting with parents of children entering the pediatric program and reevaluated this aspect of the program. The social worker was able to set up a brief intervention, focused on engaging Mr. P in JP's care, helping Mrs. P come to terms with her son's differences, and reestablishing them as a couple. Once this brief intervention was completed, the parents continued counseling at an outpatient mental health facility.

COMMENTARY

From a medical ethics perspective, the issues in rehabilitation sometimes seem to be a bit "grayer" than the norm. Most rehabilitation focuses on living with some sort of chronic illness, not trying to fix, cure, or eradicate it. The general goal is for the patient to establish a "new baseline" of functioning. So, the ethical issues are often transitional and process-oriented. Furthermore, rehabilitation care, especially rehabilitation for children, has traditionally included and considered families and significant others as active participants and even as "patients" in need of the educational and support services of the rehabilitation care team (Caplan, Callahan, Haas 1987).

It makes sense to ask in this case: Who is the patient and who should the medical system treat in order to ameliorate JP's medical issues? Is it JP, his mother, his father, the family, or the systems into which he may be integrating (the school, the CP organization)? Rehabilitation, at times, challenges the very concept of "health care." In particular, where does health care (or perhaps we should consider it "sick care" or "technology care") end and living a new and different kind of life begin? What are the roles and obligations of the rehabilitation team through this transitioning process? The treatment team and the patient and family seemed to do well until the boundaries between illness and disability began to blur. What the team views as disability or maintenance, Mrs. P views as treatment, remediation, and hope.

The case of JP highlights some of the everyday ethical dilemmas encountered by rehabilitation physicians and clinicians. The staff were able to come together and look at JP's physical and psychological needs in relationship to his family and social systems and redefine a treatment plan to address specific needs. This included requesting that Mr. and Mrs. P come together to JP's remaining treatment sessions so that they can be "on the same page" in regard to learning the "boundaries" between therapy (changing) and learning (integrating in the changes). Given the major transition into a new social and educational environment that JP was making, his parents needed guidance regarding "normal" developmental issues facing them and their son.

The parents were able to accept this developmental framework on the basis of their experience with their daughters. They needed to accept the educational transition without viewing it as the medical system abandoning them, and this was provided by the treatment team. The physiatrist's role was critical in developing this framework. The team also was able to work with the family and the school together to look at the transitional issues. Mrs. and Mr. P together were able to look at the feeding concern from this framework and agreed with the physician recommendation that this was a "medical" need and were in agreement to address it with the physician and the speech pathologist. Because the speech pathologist thought that JP would eventually be able to swallow, Mrs. P agreed to work toward that goal for the future rather than to continue to feed him solid foods currently.

In closing, we believe a cautionary note is in order. Although it is positive that the importance of the family in ethical health-care decision making is appreciated by ethicists, there is a danger that the extending of the metaphor of patient to the family can return us to the days of unwarranted paternalism. This dilemma was evident in this case at certain tension points when the treatment team was tempted to dismiss Mrs. P as "in denial." Namely, (a) when Mrs. P expressed a belief that her son could eat anything short of "tough meat" and that having him do so was worth the risk of choking and (b) when one of JP's doctors expressed the opinion that he might still benefit from certain therapies. This attitude could be seen as mere condescension. However, in this case, the particular treatment team rose above that temptation and, it seems, allowed Mrs. P to continue to make the final determination concerning what her son tried to eat. This evinces a reasonable understanding of the parent's role and still incorporates the health-care team's concerns with risks and benefits. Unless we have good reason to be suspicious, it is the parent's prerogative to interpret what is in the child's best interests within certain parameters (Buchanan and Brock 1989, 232–40; Nelson and Nelson 1995, 88–90). (Note that this mother learned the Heimlich procedure and CPR in an effort to protect her son from some of the dangers he faced in eating solid food.)

Health-care providers do well to recognize and emphasize their own fallibility, especially since it is easy for the team members to reinforce each other's thinking and cut off other view points (Purtilo 1988). Mrs. P obtains information from members of her support groups in addition to what she learns from the treatment team. The treatment team is at its best when it considers the possibility that such alternative sources of information may be reliable, and the objection should not simply be dismissed because they come from other "patients." In sum, the challenge is to continue to offer support and services to the family without always assuming that the "treatment team knows best."

REFERENCES

Allen E. Buchanan, Dan W. Brock, 1989. *Deciding for others: The ethics of surrogate decision making.* New York: Cambridge University Press.

Arthur L. Caplan, Daniel Callahan, Janet Haas, 1987. "Ethical and policy issues in rehabilitation medicine." *Hastings Center Report,* Special Supplement, 17:S1–S19.

Hilde Lindemann Nelson, James Lindemann Nelson, 1995. *The patient in the family: An ethics of medicine and families.* New York: Routledge.

Ruth B. Purtilo, 1988. "Ethical issues in teamwork: The context of rehabilitation." *Archives of Physical Medicine and Rehabilitation* 69(5):318–22.

FOR FURTHER READING

Janet Haas, 1993. "Ethical considerations of goal setting for patient care in rehabilitation medicine." *American Journal of Physical Medicine and Rehabilitation* 72(4):228–32.

Ruth B. Purtilo, 1984. "Applying the principles of informed consent to patient
care: Legal and ethical considerations for physical therapy." *Physical Therapy* 64:934–37.

Case Twenty-Six:
A New Rehab Ethics Committee
"On the Prowl"[1]

KEY TERMS: *Rehabilitation Ethics, Ethics Committees, Casuistry*

NARRATIVE

One morning, a 26-year-old man began walking the hallway between the physical therapy department (PT) and the occupational therapy department (OT) at a very rapid, determined pace. At first glance, most employees did not suspect anything amiss because outpatients often walked that hallway in a similar fashion in order to complete portions of a physical capacity test. Employees became alarmed when the man began pushing away people who were in his path.

The hospital's ethics committee was new and still "getting its feet wet" when it came to having cases referred for consultation. However, they needed to take the lead in responding to this situation of potential violence.

THE LANGUAGE AND ISSUES OF THE CASE

There were clearly several provider duties and ethical considerations that had to be honored in any solution to this situation.

> 1. The caregivers have a duty of nonmaleficence. That is, they must minimize harm. This will mean they must be concerned with the safety of the patient, the safety of other patients on the unit, and the safety of the staff. In simplest terms, this will mean that excessive force in this and similar cases must be avoided. But the question of how much force is tolerable and what procedures must be exhausted prior to the use of force to physically restrain a potentially dangerous patient is what must be determined.

---

1. This case originally appeared as Joan Nypaver and the Ethics Committee of Hillside Rehabilitation Hospital, 1996. "A new rehab ethics committee 'on the prowl.'" *Community ethics: The newsletter of the consortium ethics program* 3(3):5.

2. The caregivers should be concerned with issues of confidentiality and privacy. Although this patient's behavior was publicly observable, he was still entitled to confidentiality regarding his medical and psychiatric history. This had to be honored while explaining the situation to other concerned patients and staff who perceived a threat but were not directly involved in the patient's care.

WHAT ACTUALLY HAPPENED

Appropriate management of the situation was implemented by the staff psychologist and a member of the ethics committee. Hence, this crisis did not result in anyone being physically hurt. However, it was necessary to restrain and transfer the disturbed individual, who was in the facility for vocational treatment, to an acute care psychiatric environment.

During the debriefing that followed, which involved the participation of the facility's new ethics committee, several concerns became apparent. (a) Although the situation was handled pretty well, the ethics committee decided they needed a policy for managing potentially violent situations. (b) They decided they needed to coordinate their efforts with community resources, such as the police and rescue squad. (c) The committee members decided to create a program to educate all staff and volunteers about a safe and confidential course of action.

In identifying and beginning to address these concerns, the new ethics committee's first *official* retrospective case resolution and analysis was underway. The committee met with all interested or involved hospital employees and representatives of the police and rescue squad. They spent time discussing what went right, what could be improved, and what criteria were important in the implementation of the basic guidelines for staff and volunteers in the event of a future situation.

Next, a task force of individuals representative of the response team met and developed team functions. They outlined the priority in such a situation: de-escalating an agitated person before a situation expands into physical violence. Such a course of action recognizes the value of an individual retaining his or her autonomy by regaining self-control. They also developed educational plans for staff and volunteers in order that all would be aware of the steps taken to secure the environment, in the event of an incident, thereby allowing the team to interact with the agitated person. This strategy would eliminate voyeurism by recognizing the dignity of the agitated person, even in his compromised position.

Although the staff were unable to de-escalate the behavior of the patient in this particular case, they were able to provide some direction for his mother, who felt trapped by the fact that, although chronologically an adult, her son is not mentally competent at all times. They advised her of resources for evaluating his competency and encouraged her to share personal observations with any treatment teams, e.g., the fact that he "was agitated yesterday and this morning before leaving home" and "I tried to get him help yesterday, but his doctor would not listen to me." Thus, through the retrospective review they were able to recognize ways for this sort of situation to be avoided in the future.

This ethics committee and the task force they helped to constitute were excited about the commitment and prompt response of all parties to this case. Since then, all departments have received the hospital's Administrative Policy for "Code Red—Unruly person—potential violence" authored by the ethics committee, and they are prepared for an increasing number of case referrals.

COMMENTARY

Medical ethicists refer to case-based ethics as "casuistry." Casuists claim that ethics is primarily a matter of attention to the details or circumstances of the case. It is the details that dictate solutions (Jonsen 1991b, Kuczewski 1998a). The ethics committee at this rehabilitation hospital showed themselves to be good casuists. They were called to review a case, and they teased out the relevant considerations. They looked at what went right and what could be improved. They developed certain priorities for similar situations, e.g., de-escalating the patient's potential violence, and developed criteria concerning when stronger measures were needed. They framed generalizations about these criteria and encoded them in guidelines. Thus, they drew distinctions between cases that can be handled in one manner and other cases that demand different steps. They also noted certain considerations relevant to all these cases, e.g., avoidance of voyeurism, and took steps to educate staff concerning them. These casuists have clearly done an exemplary job.

What initially causes a particular clinical case to be labeled as an ethics case is often somewhat mysterious. But once it is identified in this way, the label sticks and a chain of events begins. This case was referred to the hospital's ethics committee because someone thought it contained ethical issues, and it did. How to insure a safe environment for patients and staff, how to detain a person humanely who threatens to harm others, how to protect his confidentiality and treat him in a way that benefits him are questions with an ethical dimension. From now on, this kind of scenario is an "ethics case" at this facility. Similar events may be referred to a different kind of administrative body at another facility, and the ethical components may not be articulated. Furthermore, new members of this ethics committee will probably be educated by the incumbent members regarding cases of this type. Such cases become a part of the "institutional conscience."

Institutional memory must be open to public scrutiny and refinement. It would seem that each rehabilitation facility would benefit from exposure to the case studies of other institutions. Through this process, each committee would become sensitive to the variety of ethical situations that can occur and would be encouraged to develop a casuistry of cases for contrasting and comparing. In this way, each hospital will be more likely to develop its institutional conscience in a more "objective" manner.

REFERENCES

Albert R. Jonsen, 1991. "Casuistry as a Methodology in Clinical Ethics." *Theoretical Medicine* 12(4):295–307.

Mark Kuczewski, 1998. "Casuistry." In Ruth Chadwick, ed. *Encyclopedia of Applied Ethics*. Vol. 1. San Diego: Academic Press, 423–32.

FOR FURTHER READING

Janet Day, Martin L. Smith, Gerald Erenberg, Robert L. Collins, 1994. "An assessment of a formal ethics committee consultation process." *HEC Forum* 6(1):18–30.

Judith Wilson Ross, John W. Glaser, Dorothy Rasinski-Gregory, Joan McIver Gibson, Corrine Bayley, 1993. *Health care ethics committees: The next generation*. American Hospital Association.

Henry J. Silverman, 1994. "Revitalizing a hospital ethics committee." *HEC Forum* 6(4):189–222.

Jacquelyn Slomka, 1994. "The ethics committee: Providing education for itself and others." *HEC Forum* 6(1):31–38.

Professional Responsibility: Employers, Colleagues, and Others

Case Twenty Seven:
Justice and Responsibility in Hiring Practices

KEY TERMS: *Equal Access, Physicians' Conflict of Interest, Justice (equal employment opportunity), Discrimination, Employers' Rights, Confidentiality, Occupational Medicine*

NARRATIVE

Ms. L, a 52-year-old woman, applied for employment as a registered nurse at a community hospital. She was scheduled for a routine pre-employment physical examination, which included a history, physical, lab work, chest X ray, and TB testing. The applicant arrived on time for her appointment. She was pale, thin, tired-looking, and seemed more nervous than the typical applicant. Her appearance was somewhat un-kempt and seemed substandard from a professional perspective.

The history provided by Ms. L. mentioned several health problems including "stomach ulcers." But this history was generally sketchy, es-pecially considering that she was a registered nurse and trained in such matters. She stated that she took iron for a while but since her hema-tocrit and hemoglobin have been normal, she no longer needs it. Ms. L did not list any previous employers but upon questioning offered the name of the hospital where she was currently employed. The inter-viewer was concerned that the applicant was attempting to be evasive or to hide something.

Upon physical examination, the physician noted no condition that would impede the applicant from discharging her prospective duties. She was cleared for hire without any limitations pending hematologic clearance. Red blood cells, hematocrit, and hemoglobin results done two days earlier were very low. Ms. L was referred to her personal phy-sician for follow-up care. Due to this referral, she was seen and admitted to the hospital from her physician's office for diagnostic evaluation of possible bleeding ulcer and for blood transfusion. The personnel de-partment at this time advised the applicant that the job offer they had tendered was now on hold until both her personal physician and the employee health physician approved of proceeding. She was advised further that she might want to reconsider resigning her present position.

Two months later, the employee health department received a no-tice that Ms. L had been medically cleared for employment by her personal physician. Nine months later, the applicant requested again to be considered for employment. She was re-examined by the same employee health physician. Her lab work results had indeed improved. The employee health physician, however, advised that she should not be hired now. He explained that the patient was hospitalized earlier that same month (discharged two weeks prior to this examination) for depression and suicidal ideation. The applicant's hospital charts were reviewed and discussed with her. Ms. L had been started on a medication called Sinequan (a sedative) which she assured him she was still taking. Ms. L was advised by the employee health physician to seek out employment in some less stressful area and to follow up regularly with her personal physician.

It is not clear to those in the personnel department why the patient wished to work at this particular hospital. Speculation among the personnel department employees ran the gamut from the fact that their hospital was near Ms. L's home to the possibility that she was "employment hopping" because of problems with her past performance. The personnel officers in charge of the case thought it better to err in the direction of caution rather than risk hiring an unstable person. They further noted that the applicant was married and did not need to work to support herself.

Ms. L's personal physician was phoned by the employee health physician and notified of the circumstances. Ms. L's personal physician felt that her physical health had improved considerably. He also believed that a job would be good rehabilitation for her and urged the employee health physician to reconsider. The applicant's treating psychiatrist was also approached by the employee health physician, and the psychiatrist also believed the patient was improving both physically and mentally.

THE LANGUAGE AND ISSUES OF THE CASE

The language of the case manifests a tension between the terms "applicant" and "patient." To Ms. L's attending physician and psychiatrist, she is a patient, and it is her best interest they are seeking. The employee health physician sees this person as a job applicant, and his main obligations are to his employer, the hospital.

The main challenge for the employee health physician and the personnel department is to treat a job applicant according to merit, qualifications, and ability to perform the job. This is the goal, and extraneous factors and speculations not directly relevant to the job must be ignored. How the patient's illness relates to her ability to perform the job must be specifically decided. Is this illness an impairment to her professional performance or would it be unfair to penalize the applicant for an irrelevant condition or a condition that would pose no problem were a "reasonable accommodation" made? If the former, then the hospital is justified in rejecting her employment application. If this condition is not directly relevant to job performance, then basing rejection of application on her health would be to discriminate unjustly and leave the hospital subject to penalties under disability related laws.

There are always confidentiality issues as well as conflict of interest issues any time a physician is the agent of an employer. Physicians normally have the best interests of the patient as their guiding aim. Serving these interests involves keeping the results of their examinations confidential, especially when the dissemination of the results is liable to victimize the patient and make her the object of prejudice. The physician in this case clearly tried to show some responsibility to the patient but had to balance this against his main obligation to his employer.

PERSPECTIVES AND KEY POINTS OF VIEW

Ms. L (the job applicant): We know precious little about her thoughts, motivations, and feelings.

Applicant's Personal Physician and Applicant's Psychiatrist: As good physicians, they have their patient's best interest at heart. They have treated her for some time and now believe that their client would benefit from this new job. They also think that the hospital is being overly cautious in its hiring practices. They believe that, as a result, the hospital is also missing out on a good employee.

These physicians also recognize an obligation to patient confidentiality. They know that certain records are important to a hirer and that these are released with the permission of their patient. In particular, the psychiatrist does not wish to divulge the explicit personal details of their psychiatric counseling sessions that he thinks are irrelevant to the hiring issue. Furthermore, given the hospital's cautiousness, it not obvious that more information would help his patient to be hired.

Employee Health Physician: He does not believe he has any real responsibilities to the job applicant he examined other than to refer her for treatment for immanent conditions. Ms. L is not his patient. Usually he talks about how important it is to vulnerable patients in the hospital that they only be cared for "by the best." Being a health-care professional at this hospital is a privilege, not a right, and only the fittest merit the privilege. This sentiment is lauded by his employer, the hospital.

Personnel Department Staff: Their attitude is similar to that of the employee health physician. However, it is also fairly clear from their speculations that they "blame" the job applicant for continuing to pose a problem for them. They wish she'd go back to her old job and not continue to seek review of her application for employment.

WHAT ACTUALLY HAPPENED

Despite the recommendations of the applicant's personal physician and her psychiatrist, the employee health physician nonetheless decided that in view of the hospital's primary mission to serve its patients, he could not recommend hiring the applicant. The employee health physician personally called the applicant at her home and advised her of his recommendation. The hospital followed his recommendation and did not hire the applicant.

We now have additional facts based upon the hindsight afforded by the passage of a couple of years. The applicant has been seen as a patient in the emergency room or hospitalized at this facility several times (nine), mostly for gastrointestinal problems. It is not known if the patient presently is employed. She lists herself as an agency nurse.

COMMENTARY

The hospital, like any employer, has an ethical and legal obligation not to discriminate against people because of social factors or personal characteristics that are not directly relevant to their job performance. Although it is a typical maxim of ethics that we should treat persons as ends-in-themselves rather than simply as means, professional roles demand that we evaluate the person objectively regarding his or her ability to carry out the duties specific to the role. This is the crux of the matter. Is this person capable of carrying out her duties at the time of the initial interview? Currently?

There is no clear-cut answer to this question. However, it is important that those in responsibility stick to what is known about the applicant at the time they are passing the judgment. An offer is tendered to this person that is withdrawn due to the need to treat her ulcer. It is possible that the main reason this nurse is rejected by a hospital sorely in need of nursing staff (as evidenced by the haste with which the initial offer was made) is that they may not wish to add her pre-existing conditions to their insurance situation (Pear 1993). Furthermore, speculation regarding the relationship between her marital status and her financial need indicates stereotyping and can be indicative of discrimination by the personnel department.

Furthermore, much discussion can focus on the relationship between nondiscrimination and professionalism. On the one hand, we do not wish to take into account personal qualities that do not affect job performance. On the other hand, the concept of a profession is one that differs from a mere job. A job is what one does for pay, but ideally a profession involves who one is and one's way of being. Thus, it may establish certain standards to be met, which do not immediately translate into the performance of a specific task.

But we must be careful not to exaggerate the requirements of a job or profession or fail to appreciate the mechanisms that have been developed to monitor and improve such situations regarding new hires (e.g., probation periods that follow after hiring, periodic performance reviews), or underestimate the back-up systems that exist for dealing with illness or instability in a team member. It is too easy to think of one's profession as requiring perfection and to react harshly to deviations from the norm. In this way, the employee health physician and personnel department staff were probably unjust in denying a position to a person who was qualified.

Also worth noting is that the employee health staff seem to know a good deal about the episodes when Ms. L was subsequently treated at their hospital. This is one of those unfortunate breaches of patient confidentiality that is so common within the health-care system.

FOR FURTHER READING

Sue Gena Lurie, 1994. "Ethical dilemmas and professional roles in occupational medicine." *Social Science and Medicine* 38(10): 1367–74.

Robert Pear, 1993. "The disabled gain new rights to jobs and health insurance; 'Equal Access' ruling affects millions in U.S." *New York Times* June 9, A1, A10.

Stephen E. Toulmin, 1986. "Divided loyalties and ambiguous relationships." *Social Science and Medicine* 23(8): 783–87.

Diana Chapman Walsh, 1986. "Divided loyalties in medicine: The ambivalence of occupational medical practice." *Social Science and Medicine* 23(8): 789–96.

Case Twenty-Eight:
Conflicts among Physicians: Playing "Resident in the Middle"

Players:

Mrs. P (the Patient)
Mr. P (the Patient's Husband)
Dr. Reed (the Resident)
Dr. Stevens (the "On-Call" Surgeon)

Dr. Gibson (the Consulting Gastroenterologist)
Dr. Perkins (the Consulting Pulmonologist)

KEY TERMS: *Physician Conflicts, Informed Consent, Medical Uncertainty*

NARRATIVE

Mrs. P was a 30-year-old married woman with two children. She presented with a two-week history of low-grade fever (101 degrees), upper right quadrant pain, and right lower chest pain. Her initial exam by the resident (Dr. Reed) was normal except for the low-grade fever. No specific diagnosis was made, and she was sent home.

Mrs. P failed to improve, and she was again seen in a few days. Again, her exam was normal except for fever. A battery of tests were done, revealing an elevated white count, elevated liver function, a slight lower lobe infiltrate, and gallstones. The presumptive diagnosis was right lower lobe pneumonia and coincident gallstones. She was placed on antibiotics and sent home. Within 24 hours her condition worsened, and she presented to the emergency room with fever (103 degrees), severe right upper quandrant pain radiating to the right and the supraclavicular area. She was mildly short of breath and very frightened.

Her husband accompanied Mrs. P to the emergency room (ER), and he was angry because she had gotten worse despite therapy. He demanded immediate answers to his questions and spoke in a loud and occasionally vulgar manner. Mrs. P, in contrast, was a rather passive, soft-spoken individual. She asked few questions, never proffered an opinion, and simply expressed that she wanted to get better. She accepted the advice and actions of her husband and physicians unquestioningly.

On Dr. Reed's exam in the ER, the patient manifested heightened tenderness in the right upper quadrant with guarding. Her lab tests had also worsened. It was suspected that she had acute cholecystitis (an inflammation of the gallbladder) with a sympathetic pleural reaction rather than pneumonia. Dr. Stevens, the on-call surgeon, was consulted. He examined Mrs. P in a hasty and abrupt manner that seemed to exacerbate her pain and anger her husband. Dr. Stevens stated that Mrs. P needed to be admitted, given IV antibiotics, and to receive her nutrition via a nasogastric tube. Dr. Stevens requested that Dr. Reed serve as the admitting physician, and he would act as the consultant.

Dr. Stevens's recommendations were carried out, but Mrs. P failed to improve immediately. She seemed to become more frightened about her condition and Mr. P became still more hostile. He complained about the lack of improvement, the nasogastric tube, and the surgeon's manner. Mr. P's demeanor and his manner of expressing these complaints alienated virtually all who interacted with him.

After one day of hospitalization, Mrs. P's condition did not improve, and Dr. Stevens believed that surgery was necessary to remove the gallstones. Mr. P refused and wanted a second opinion. Dr. Reed discussed the case with the attending faculty member, who showed no interest in the case and who did not interview or examine the patient. The faculty member suggested that a gastroenterologist, Dr. Gibson, be consulted. Dr. Gibson was unable to confirm or rule out the diagnosis on the basis of his examination. He suggested further observation because the patient's condition had not deteriorated. This recommendation appeased Mr. P but angered Dr. Stevens.

The following day, a Friday, the patient was still no better and stated that she had vomited blood. Dr. Reed believed that this was due to stress and the nasogastric tube. Dr. Gibson, the gastroenterologist, interpreted this event as coughing up blood and therefore believed the patient had a pulmonary embolus (PE). A ventilation/perfusion scan was done, and the results indicated low probability of pulmonary embolus. Nevertheless, Dr. Gibson held firm to his diagnosis while Dr. Stevens continued to believe that Mrs. P needed surgery. Dr. Reed encouraged Dr. Stevens to discuss his views directly with Dr. Gibson. Dr. Gibson subsequently called Dr. Reed to say that he could not reason with Dr. Stevens and that he was signing himself off the case because he did not believe the patient to have a gastroenterologic problem. Dr. Reed then called Dr. Perkins, a pulmonologist, for a consultation.

Before the pulmonologist could examine the patient, Dr. Stevens procured the patient's consent to surgery. The patient was taken to the operating room at about 4:00 P.M. and prepped for surgery. However, Mr. P arrived at the hospital at about this time and demanded that the operation not take place. Dr. Stevens was, of course, furious and called Dr. Reed saying that he, too, was signing off the case because of the difficulty of dealing with Mr. P.

THE LANGUAGE AND ISSUES OF THE CASE

Clearly the word "conflict" comes to mind when reading this case. As is often the case in large hospitals with residency programs, many physicians are involved in this situation, and one almost needs a scorecard to keep track of them. But one cannot stop at the mere identification of conflict. It is important to find the causes of conflict and to highlight the values being compromised by the conflict. Some lines of question worth pursuing might include the following:

1. Were the patient's wishes and concerns respected?
2. Did all physicians act according to reasonable ideals of professional conduct?
3. Did the patient's husband act in a reasonable manner? Ethically speaking, did he have any real rights as a decision maker? Did he, at any point, forfeit those rights?
4. In what relationship do the physicians stand to each other? What constitutes reasonable expectations in the multiple physician-patient relationships? When is it appropriate to terminate the relationship and on what grounds?
5. What constitutes reasonable expectations in the physician-family relationship? What is the physician's obligation to involve the husband in decision making?
6. Was an informed consent for surgery actually obtained in this case? What constitutes informed consent and were its elements present in the consent for surgery? What information needed to be communicated to the patient/family for the fulfillment of the requirements of informed consent?

WHAT ACTUALLY HAPPENED

The patient was returned to her room, and Dr. Perkins, the pulmonologist, had the opportunity to examine her. He confirmed a diagnosis of pulmonary embolism. The patient was treated appropriately and recovered normally. The patient's response to therapy allayed the fears of Mr. and Mrs. P and no further conflicts occurred with the physicians or hospital staff.

COMMENTARY

There were several stumbling blocks to the adequate care of Mrs. P. Certainly the patient, a shy person who was clearly intimidated by her husband and the physicians, could not easily exercise her autonomy given the heated conflict among the staff members. The resident who was trapped in the middle of the conflict was inexperienced and found it difficult to manage the interpersonal conflicts and deal effectively with the diagnostic uncertainty. This is a tragically common situation (Shreves and Moss 1996). It is the uncertainty and the resulting conflicts that dominate the narrative. Ironically, the physicians and the patient's husband all believed they were merely attending to the medical facts. That is, they acted like characters in a story that involves making the correct diagnosis, prescribing a course of treatment, and sending a healthy or recovering patient home again. The repeated failure of the narrative to resemble anything like this medical model does not deter the characters from continuing to play those roles in a self-righteous manner.

The usual conception of informed consent also works on the medical model of diagnosis, treatment, and cure. The physician makes the diagnosis, proposes a treatment and alternatives, explains the risks and benefits, and receives authorization from the patient, or treatment is refused. In this approach, informed consent is a one-time event that is played out immediately before treatment. Clearly Dr. Stevens, the on-call surgeon, continued to force the narrative into this model up to the point where Mr. P derailed the surgery. This model of the medical narrative and the role of informed consent does not fit very well in cases of medical uncertainty. Where diagnosis, prognosis, and treatment are unclear, this model of informed consent seems ludicrous.

Typically, health-care providers attempt to portray confidence in their diagnosis and proposed treatment to the patient and family and do not adequately convey the element of uncertainty (Katz 1984a, 165–206; Katz 1984b; Fox 1980). Or they do not admit their uncertainty because they fail to realize that their diagnostic knowledge is of a hypothetical and constructivist nature (Hunter 1991, 1996). Either way, the failure to share uncertainty can lead to anger by the patient and family when events do not go as had been forecast by the professionals. Although this seemed to be the case here, the physicians, particularly Dr. Stevens, still continued to portray their diagnoses as sure-footed and certain.

It seems that in this situation the physicians only perceived two options regarding informed consent: (a) portray the diagnosis as certain and proceed with informed consent as usual or (b) cease discussing the case with Mr. and Mrs. P because the couple are not physicians and so cannot understand the situation. Clearly, there is a third alternative. Namely, they could provide information regarding the indeterminacy of their diagnoses and explain whatever plan they could mutually devise to arrive at greater certainty. In this way, they would not be providing information merely to enable the Ps to make a choice but would be conceiving of autonomy as respect, as a person's desire to know what is going on. The Ps needed to be reassured that those in charge cared about the problem and were taking steps to resolve it.

Physicians are often reluctant to convey uncertainty, fearing they will heighten the anxiety of the patient and family. Mr. P's reactions indicate just the opposite— the feeling that information was being withheld led to greater suspicion and hostility than conveying uncertainty might have. To see autonomy in terms of respect for the patient's need to understand her condition and know what is happening in her environment is to see informed consent as a process (Lidz, Appelbaum, Meisel 1988) that tries to make "transparent" the thinking of the physician to the patient (Brody 1989).

On a pragmatic and bureaucratic level, the problem of this case can also be interpreted in terms of the difficult position in which a young resident was placed in having to manage the competing specialists. The specialists were seeing the illness through their particular lenses. The resident was too inexperienced and lacked the power to be an effective advocate for the patient even though he was institutionally positioned to fill the role that one's primary care or family physician often does as "captain of the team." It is questionable whether a resident should be in such a position in a difficult case, and if so, more formalized mechanisms for dealing with attending physicians and consultants must be created (Shreves and Moss 1996; Council on Ethical and Judicial Affairs 1994). The attending faculty member should have become more involved, and the resident should perhaps have made an additional appeal to him. It is extremely important that someone, the resident or the attending faculty member, explain each of these steps to the patient and husband during the attempt to secure a diagnosis so that the family does not feel abandoned.

If an orderly plan of treatment could not be secured through the attending faculty member, Dr. Reed, the resident, could have engaged the services of the medical staff director or department head. Someone in a position of authority could have been consulted to evaluate the situation and keep the physicians in line with proper medical etiquette. The resident, as a person in a subservient position, obviously feared that he would be perceived as incompetent if he were seen by these authorities as "making a big deal out of nothing." This possibility is real and often forms the background in clinical "turf wars." Negotiating these conflicts in a satisfactory way that does not villainize others is a political skill that is often at the heart of practice in today's large health-care institutions, particularly academic institutions and teaching hospitals.

REFERENCES

Howard Brody, 1989. "Transparency: Informed consent in primary care." *Hastings Center Report* 19(5):5–9.

Council on Ethical and Judicial Affairs, American Medical Association, 1994. "Disputes between medical supervisors and trainees." *Journal of the American Medical Association* 272(23):1861–65.

Jay Katz, 1984a. *The silent world of doctor and patient.* New York: Free Press.

———1984b. "Why doctors don't disclose uncertainty." *Hastings Center Report* 14(1):35–44.

Renee C. Fox, 1980. "The evolution of medical uncertainty." *Milbank Memorial Fund Quarterly* 58(1):1–49.

Kathryn Montgomery Hunter, 1991. *Doctors' stories: The narrative structure of medical knowledge.* Princeton, NJ: Princeton University Press.

———1996. "Narrative, literature, and the clinical exercise of practical reason." *Journal of Medicine and Philosophy* 21(3): 303–20.

Charles W. Lidz, Paul S. Appelbaum, Alan Meisel, 1988. "Two models of implementing informed consent." *Archives of Internal Medicine* 148:1385–89.

Jennifer Giaquinto Shreves, Alvin H. Moss, 1996. "Residents' ethical disagreements with attending physicians: An unrecognized problem." *Academic Medicine* 71(10):1103–1105.

FOR FURTHER READING

Mark J. DiNubile, 1990. "Responsibility for patient care: Where does the buck stop?" *American Journal of Medicine* 88(4):405–406.

Case Twenty-Nine:
In Whose Interest? Withholding the Truth
from a Patient

KEY TERMS: *Truth Telling, Lying, Informed Consent, Competence, Decision-Making Capacity, Surrogate Decision Making, Therapeutic Privilege*

NARRATIVE

Ms. Q was a 72-year-old widowed woman who currently lived with her daughter. Her past history was significant for the development of a major depression several years before, which developed after the death of a handicapped younger brother who had been under Ms. Q's care since the death of their parents. Also significant in her past history was a bout with rectal cancer.

The cancer had penetrated through the walls of the bowel and involved local lymph nodes; however, the tumor was entirely removed at the time of surgery. As was then considered standard therapy, Ms. Q was begun on a postoperative course of radiation and chemotherapy. The patient, however, had a great deal of reluctance about starting the chemotherapy and radiation therapy but did so at her daughter's request. During the course of that therapy, the patient had a massive myocardial infarction (MI) which, according to her cardiologist, resulted in extremely poor heart function. Her physicians believed that Ms. Q had a very limited life expectancy on the basis of this heart disease. She never completed the chemotherapy and radiation therapy because of the very long recuperative period that was necessary after her MI.

Over the course of the last six months, Ms. Q was discovered to have developed evidence of bilateral lung masses on chest X-ray. These were presumed to be metastases from her previous rectal carcinoma. Notes in the medical record indicate that this diagnosis was discussed with Mrs. Q's daughter and that she did not wish the patient to be informed of it. Because of the patient's heart disease and generally weakened condition, the daughter did not want her mother to receive any further cancer treatments. The patient was under the care of a surgeon at this time who was the physician involved in this decision.

Ms. Q was recently hospitalized in the psychiatry unit on the advice of her surgeon because of severe depression. The psychiatrist's notes indicated that the interaction of the patient with her daughter showed the daughter to be protective of Mrs. Q but with very limited insight as to her mother's treatment needs, particularly concerning her depression. The patient's daughter expressed the feeling that her mother would not, and could not, improve with psychiatric intervention. The patient herself was disinterested in the question of whether she would like to stay in the hospital for treatment or be discharged to her home. Her daughter continued to advocate for the patient to be discharged to her home.

At this time, Ms. Q began to complain of a cough and some anterior chest discomfort, probably caused by her pulmonary metastases. The cough was not very severe, and she did not appear to be having any great discomfort or any shortness of breath. Oncology consultation was requested regarding the need for bronchoscopy, for possible diagnostic biopsy, and to advise whether any role for radiation or chemotherapy was needed.

The oncologists, psychiatrists, and house staff were informed that the patient's daughter had expressed very strong wishes that they not speak with Mrs. Q regarding the diagnosis of apparent metastatic cancer or regarding the need to find out if the patient was capable of making decisions about her medical care. Paradoxically, Ms. Q's daughter, on at least one occasion, spoke openly in front of the patient concerning her abnormal chest X ray and possible radiation or chemotherapy. The daughter finally assented to allowing the oncologists to examine her mother and discuss the situation with the patient.

Conversations between the house staff and Ms. Q took place over several days. Initially the patient seemed to wish to know more about her medical condition and continued to express interest even after being asked if she would want to know about "bad news." She subsequently added that her chief wish was just to die soon. On another occasion, Ms. Q was asked questions about her prior bowel surgery, radiation treatments, and chemotherapy. She was unable to recall ever having had bowel surgery and specifically did not recall ever being told anything about having cancer or a tumor. She did not recall having had radiation or chemotherapy. Ms. Q seemed quite apathetic and appeared to have no real interests when asked about television programs, hobbies, or things she liked to do. Neurological and psychological testing indicated that the patient suffered from mild to moderate dementia.

THE LANGUAGE AND ISSUES OF THE CASE

Cases of withholding the truth from patients tend to suggest the classic language and dichotomies of medical ethics, such as lying versus truth-telling and respect for the patient's autonomy versus the duty not to inflict harm on the patient (nonmaleficence). But such dichotomies do not get us anywhere in and of themselves. We must answer certain basic questions.

1. Should requests to withhold information like the one that Ms. Q's daughter made be honored? If so, under what circumstances?
2. Should Ms. Q continue to be informed of her condition and changes in it?
3. Should the patient continue to be involved in the decision-making process? Is she competent to be involved in the process of informed consent or treatment refusal? If not, are there reasons to continue to pass along information to her?

PERSPECTIVES AND KEY POINTS OF VIEW

The Surgeon, the Cardiologist, and the Patient's Daughter: The patient's surgeon agreed with the daughter for several years that the patient was not competent to decide her own affairs, and they had formed a partnership in withholding information. The cardiologist had also explicitly told the patient's daughter that he supported her actions in not informing Ms. Q of the possibility of recurrent cancer. He felt that the addition of more depressing and burdensome information would place great stress on Ms. Q and that it was quite possible that this would seriously worsen her condition. All three of these persons took up a position as beneficent protectors of the patient, who thought they were preventing her from receiving information that would cause sadness or alarm.

The Psychiatrist and Oncologist: During the hospital admission that formed the basis of this presentation, the psychiatrist was the attending physician. He was trying to treat the patient for depression and ran into considerable opposition from the patient's daughter, who felt that such treatment was either unnecessary or unlikely to be helpful or some combination of the two.

Both the psychiatrist and the consulting oncologist questioned whether Ms. Q should be excluded from the decision-making process and worried that a great deal of her disorientation owed to medical tests and treatments without any explanation being given to her concerning the diagnosis and treatment process.

Ms. Q: It is very difficult to know this person's viewpoint, particularly because she had long been in a dependent and uninformed situation by the time anyone sought to explore her wishes. At that point, she was depressed and suffering from mental impairment, presumably a complication from her MI. It is not clear how much "keeping her in the dark" contributed to her condition. It is possible that Ms. Q was often confused by the treatments and medical tests she received along the way without benefit of explanation. This certainly can contribute to a loss of a sense of agency and add to depression. However, this is, of necessity, conjecture.

WHAT ACTUALLY HAPPENED

The patient's cardiologist indicated that her heart condition was so poor that the risk of bronchoscopy even for diagnostic purposes was considered excessive. Possible treatment of the pulmonary masses with radiation was also deemed to pose excessive risks. Ms. Q, after several more days of hospitalization for treatment of her depression, was discharged to the care of her daughter.

COMMENTARY

This case is extraordinary in the way it raises the issue of "respect" for persons and the doctrine of informed consent. Much of the literature on informed consent revolves around the patient's right of self-determination and the value of patient autonomy. The implication of such an emphasis is that we wish to allow the person to make choices. Conversely, if there are few choices to be made, we may wonder about the need to inform the patient. Hence, it seems foolhardy to attempt to persuade families to tell patients news the family is not convinced the patient wants.

Nevertheless, the erosion of the general principles and the ethos that should govern the doctor-patient relationship is at stake in this type of case. Although autonomy and choice are important, autonomy can also be thought of as an expression of respect for the person. Paternalism is bad not only because it violates patient autonomy, but because it violates an ethic of respecting the patient as a mature, free human being who is entitled to be aware of his or her own affairs. Even when people do not desire to be the "managers" of their health care, they often desire to know all the relevant information (Lidz, Meisel, et al. 1983; Meisel and Kuczewski 1996). Seldom is this information harmful in the long run but it often restores a sense of agency (Sheldon 1982; Bok 1978, 232–55). One should be wary of claims that information would be harmful to the patient (a claim of "therapeutic privilege") without good reason for believing so (President's Commission 1982, 95–96).

This case also calls our attention to another related point. Namely, informed consent is a process, and so is lying. At some point, someone withholds the truth from a patient. Another person implicitly or explicitly joins in the deception. Soon, the patient is being denied information by all involved in her care. Of course, as we've seen at points in this case, vigilance in deception may occasionally wane. But such lapses matter little because the process of deception has its own momentum and all parties, sometimes including the patient, abide by implicit established norms with regard to the exchange of information. The process of deception can be very difficult to reverse. As we saw in this case, past a certain point, it can be near impossible to do so effectively.

REFERENCES

Sisela Bok, 1978. *Lying: Moral choice in public and private life.* New York: Pantheon Books.

Charles W. Lidz, Alan Meisel, Marian Osterweis, Janice L. Holden, John H. Marx, Mark R. Munetz, 1983. "Barriers to informed consent." *Annals of Internal Medicine* 99(4):539–43.

Alan Meisel, Mark Kuczewski, 1996. "Legal and ethical myths about informed consent." *Archives of Internal Medicine* 156:2521–26.

President's Commission for the Study of Ethical Problems in Medicine and Biomedical and Behavioral Research, 1982. *Making health care decisions,* Vol. 1, Washington, DC: U.S. Government Printing Office.

Mark Sheldon, 1982. "Truth telling in medicine." *Journal of the American Medical Association* 247(5):651–54.

FOR FURTHER READING

Dennis Novack, Barbara Detering, Robert Arnold, Lachlan Forrow, Morissa Ladinsky, John Pezzullo, 1989. "Physicians' attitudes toward using deception to resolve difficult ethical problems." *Journal of the American Medical Association* 261(20):2980–85.

AIDS: Problems of Confidentiality

Case Thirty:
Confidentiality and Caring

KEY TERMS: *Confidentiality, Futility, Religion in Medical Decision Making*

NARRATIVE

Howard was a 33-year-old man admitted to the hospice program several months ago with an admitting diagnosis of AIDS (end stage). Born in Israel, he emigrated to the United States fifteen years before in order to enter an Orthodox Jewish rabbinical school. When a routine blood test revealed that he was HIV positive, Howard and his teachers mutually decided that he leave his New York City school and community. He then came to Cleveland knowing no one and keeping his HIV status a complete secret for eight years. Prior to getting sick (about two years ago) he was active as an artist working in a frame shop. For fun, he liked to go to Jewish folk dances and socialize with friends. Even though Howard was not active in the Cleveland religious community, his life revolved around his heritage and strict religious beliefs.

For a man like Howard, illness was a heavy burden. The hospice admitting nurse noted:

> "Pt. lives alone. Family lives in Israel and doesn't know of illness at pt.'s request; feels that they would be shamed, (has not seen family for 17 years since he left Israel). Pt. with many conflicts regarding family, illness, identity, religion. Private man has trouble asking for and receiving help. Support available through religious community."

During the intake visit he also indicated in regard to future pain control, that he "does not want to be drowsy, wants to be able to pray. I'm a fighter, I'm not giving up."

Once diagnosed with AIDS, Howard formed alliances with a Cleveland civic group (the Cleveland AIDS Task Force), a local Jewish community in a nearby neighborhood, and this hospice program. Nurses arranged monthly meetings with the Jewish Family Services to discuss and coordinate all available care. Present at these meetings were social workers, representatives from the CATF, and rabbis from the Orthodox community. The group discussed the difficulty of finding volunteers because of Howard's hesitancy to accept help, especially from those of different cultural and religious backgrounds. Fear of rejection and a desire to keep his diagnosis a secret complicated the community's effort to help. Even though Howard was independent at the beginning of his hospice association, he did not have a constant caretaker available for when things worsened. Plans for him to move to the neighborhood in which there was a larger Jewish community in order to be closer to his caretakers did not come to fruition.

Despite frequent hospitalization (fever, herpes, wasting, pneumonia) during his hospice association, Howard wished to have all extraordinary measures performed. Three months after entering the hospice program, Howard still wanted full code status. During the next two months, the hospice social worker met often with him to explore options concerning long-term skilled nursing care in a nursing facility. The application forms required that Howard be asked about tube feedings, CPR, etc., and Howard "became withdrawn and nervous." A rabbi friend was designated as his surrogate on his durable power of attorney for health care (DPAHC) and would make decisions for Howard should he become incapable of speaking for himself. Together they discussed advance directives and consulted the Rabbinical Association in New York for information and direction.

There was much to sort out in making the advance directives. Since Howard believed he got AIDS because he "was bad" and it was a justifiable punishment from God, he feared facing Him. Religiously, he perceived that every minute on earth was to be used in order to make the world a holy place. Doing his work "here" was very important. Advice obtained from the religious authority encouraged the full code status. Empathy was given by the rabbis but was mingled with strictness and little comfort. It was difficult for the hospice workers to sort out completely what Howard imposed on himself and what was imposed by religious authority.

At Howard's last home visit, his primary hospice nurse, visiting, found him to be dehydrated due to scant PO (i.e., through the mouth) intake, and the apartment temperature on that hot summer day was 120 degrees. Knowing he would die if left alone, she called the paramedics. Upon their arrival, his HIV and code status were discussed with them. They were very upset with this information and treated the patient roughly despite his severe pain. The nurse was not sure that his wishes would have been respected had he arrested in the ambulance.

The subsequent hospital admission brought the DNR decision to a head. Howard's condition had deteriorated, and his primary physician was getting direction from the patient's HMO that a continued hospital stay was inappropriate. Howard was fully oriented but in a great deal of pain. (Due to Kaposi sarcoma, he had multiple open lesions, with 4+ edema of his trunk and lower extremities.) The primary physician contacted the hospice to see if they could influence Howard to forgo life-prolonging measures such as a feeding tube and CPR. If Howard did so, it would greatly enhance his chances of admission to the hospice in-patient unit (IPU). Ironically, when the home hospice nurse made a friendly visit a couple of days later, Howard initiated the DNR topic. Due to his deteriorating condition and with the support of his rabbi, he no longer wanted life support. He signed a DNR statement. It was noted on the form that the "patient hopes for good health, but is simply accepting the seriousness of his condition." He was admitted to the hospice IPU.

While on the unit, a person from CATF called Howard's brother in Israel and without telling Howard informed the brother of the situation. Evidently, this CATF person and some members of the local religious community felt that this was Howard's unspoken wish. Earlier, Howard had ceremoniously packed all his belongings and sent them to his family in Israel. The rabbi felt this may have indicated that the patient was symbolically mailing himself home and putting closure to a stage of his struggles. When his brother arrived, Howard was surprised and voiced some unhappiness that he had not been consulted. They then spent much time talking and shared some kosher dinners. Howard's 29-year-old brother then spent a night on the unit and helped to care for his sibling.

It was then Howard's brother who decided (with much soul searching and consultation) to inform his father of the patient's condition. The two of them then decided to tell the mother that Howard had skin cancer, for she would be too ashamed to walk through her town if the real diagnosis were known. The parents quickly flew to New York and then on to Cleveland. Howard was awake when they arrived. His mother was crying and saying, "My son, my son," and his father's look was one of devastation. The primary hospice nurse, who had come to be very trusted by Howard, taught the parents how to administer water with a syringe for thirst as well as other comfort measures. They performed all tasks lovingly while touching their son. He died approximately five hours later with them at his side. The family flew Howard's body back to Israel.

THE LANGUAGE AND ISSUES OF THE CASE

This case clearly raises issues of confidentiality. In particular, it pits the duty to respect a patient's privacy against the caregivers' desire to violate confidentiality in an effort to help the patient (beneficence) and to meet his social needs. As we saw, the caregivers believe they were re-

specting an "unspoken wish" and therefore still respecting their patient's autonomy. However, not requiring wishes to be spoken clearly
raises certain problems.

PERSPECTIVES AND KEY POINTS OF VIEW

The Hospice Nurse: She had a good sense of Howard's struggle
with the guilt over contracting his illness and his effort to use his suffering to reconcile himself to his spiritual beliefs. However, (a) she wished
to see Howard receive the level of care he needed. And (b) she wished to
facilitate his processing of his guilt as quickly as possible. Otherwise,
Howard's time on earth might elapse before he had a chance to do
things such as say good-bye to his family. Therefore, she also understood the desire of some of Howard's friends to "take things into their
own hands."

Howard: Howard was clearly a person who loved life but also
was suffering greatly. He believed his illness stemmed from his wrong-
doing, but it also contained the possibility of redemption. Nevertheless,
he did not wish to suffer more than was necessary. But he had to rely
on the interpretation of authorities regarding decisions about limiting
his suffering. He felt that his transgressions had disqualified him as an
interpreter of the law in regard to his situation.

COMMENTARY

Our society values religious freedom. As such, we must allow people
to express their religious values in their end-of-life decisions. This is a
legal and moral principle with which few disagree. However, this case
shows that in the lived realities of an ongoing care-giving relationship,
the boundaries between persons are somewhat fluid, and there is an
interaction of values among the parties. Thus the care-giving relationship becomes one of mutual self-discovery (Kuczewski 1996, 34–35).

The hospice nurse was able to respect the patient's wishes—i.e., for
full code status—throughout the process. But it was certainly clear to
the patient that this nurse had certain beliefs regarding what would be
best for him even if she respected their differences. And the patient
eventually came to reconcile his beliefs with the preferences held by the
nurse for forgoing treatment. There is nothing wrong with this kind of
decision-making intimacy. In fact, it truly shows the ideal of informed
consent as shared decision making.

However, one has to be careful. Just because caregivers become
closely involved in the patient's decision-making process does not nul-

lify all boundaries and considerations of a patient's rights. This is shown by the call the person from the Cleveland task force placed to the patient's brother. This person did this as a friend, but even for a friend, it is still a questionable call. Had a health-care worker done it without the assent of the patient, she would have clearly violated normal considerations of confidentiality.[1] One can certainly produce humane and humanistic reasons for crossing this boundary, and it may even be that the results are quite good in any individual case. However, such consequentialist considerations cannot hold sway. Ultimately, we must be deontologists in regard to violating a patient's confidentiality. Health-care professionals simply cannot assume they know best, even if they know the patient well. Mutual self-discovery is about a dialogue between patient and provider, not about a return to paternalism.

Of course, this confidence is not broken for any of the usual reasons associated with AIDS. Typically, we debate the provider's duty to break confidentiality in order to warn contacts of the patient about the possibility of infection from a consensual sexual contact (Bayer 1996a), from a coerced sexual contact (Bayer 1996b), or from seeking treatment from an infected health-care provider (Gostin 1991). Similarly, we debate the mandatory determination of HIV status when there is a good chance that treatment will avoid the spread of the disease (Bayer 1995). And, of course, we are always concerned when violations of confidentiality will result in discrimination against an infected person (Gostin 1997). Note that in each of these cases, the interests of some party—e.g., an insurer, a partner, a victim, or a child—is pitted against that of an HIV-infected patient. As a result, we are very cautious about confidentiality and require justification for it. In the case at hand, no one's interests are pitted against Howard's. So, even though we might wish that Howard's assent had been obtained before breaking his confidence, we tend to be sympathetic to this person since she was clearly trying to act in his best interest alone.

In general, however, this case is a testimony to "care giving." Those involved in patient care genuinely treated the whole patient throughout the illness and were willing to renegotiate plans as the situation changed. The energy and stamina this must have taken are enormous. But, one can sense from the tone of the case report that those involved

---

1. By "assent," we mean that this need not be phrased as a question. The nurse could have told Howard, "I think it is time to call your family. I feel I must contact your brother." This would have given him an opportunity to react if he still felt strongly that his confidentiality should not be violated.

were edified by their efforts. This is the part of the self-discovery that the provider undergoes.

REFERENCES

Ronald Bayer, 1995. "Women's rights, babies' interests: Ethics, politics, and science in the debate of newborn HIV screening." In H. L. Minkoff, J. A. De-Hovitz, A. Duerr, eds. *HIV infection in women*. New York:Raven Press, 293–307.

Ronald Bayer, 1996a. "AIDS prevention—Sexual ethics and responsibility." *New England Journal of Medicine* 334(23):1540–42.

Ronald Bayer, 1996b. "When victims need to know: Sometimes it's O.K. to test the accused for HIV." *New York Times*: A23, Jan 18.

Lawrence Gostin, 1991. "The HIV-infected health care professional: Public policy, discrimination, and patient safety." *Archives of Internal Medicine* 151(4): 663–65.

Lawrence Gostin, 1997. "Health care information and the protection of personal privacy: Ethical and legal considerations." *Annals of Internal Medicine* 127 (8, Pt.2):683–90.

Mark Kuczewski, 1996. "Reconceiving the family: The process of consent in medical decisionmaking." *Hastings Center Report* 26(2):30–37

Case Thirty-One:
Confidentiality and the Duty to Warn

KEY TERMS: *Confidentiality, Duty to Warn, AIDS*

NARRATIVE

Erica, a newborn white female, was referred to a hospital-based pediatric HIV clinic for evaluation of perinatal exposure to maternal HIV infection. The mother, 21-year-old Ms. X, was tested postnatally after a needle-stick accident sustained by hospital personnel. (According to the referring physician, Ms. X was presented with this information, and the implications for herself and infant were discussed at length. She was given clear directions for both pediatric and self follow-up medical care).

Over the next three months, the physician and social worker at the children's hospital made numerous attempts to locate the mother and schedule pediatric HIV testing and to insure that the infant received Bacitrim for pneumocystis carinii pneumonia (PCP) prophylaxis. They left numerous messages with a friend whose telephone number was the only one Ms. X listed on prenatal admission, they mailed letters, mailed certified letters, had the police go to her home and told her to contact the doctor at the hospital for an appointment, and finally contacted Children and Youth Services (CYS) for assistance. CYS had not made contact with Ms. X.

Erica presented at a local pediatrician's office for treatment of her diaper rash. The pediatrician prevailed upon the mother to take the baby to the hospital for HIV testing. And Ms. X did so.

At the hospital appointment, Ms. X appeared with the baby's father, James, but had him stay in the waiting room. Ms. X did not want him to know her HIV status or the nature of their child's visit to the hospital. She did not believe James to be the source of her HIV infection and was apprehensive about his reaction should he learn of her diagnosis. Ms. X also revealed during this first visit that although she and James had been living together until one week prior to visit, she had moved out after an argument and was now living with a male friend, Hubert. She insisted that this was strictly platonic and Hubert was merely. "helping her out."

Ms. X was strongly encouraged to notify James of the situation and encourage him to be tested. The physician and social worker offered to

187

assist with this process if Ms. X felt it would be helpful. She expressed her intention to make this disclosure in the future, but was not ready to do so at this time. Ms. X was also provided with information about safe sex practices, but she vigorously denied being sexually active. At appointment's end, the physician spoke with James about the visit, informing him that there were concerns about the adequacy of the baby's immune system to fight off infection.

Over the next four months Erica was followed at this hospital, usually with a pattern of one or two missed appointments before one was kept. Erica's HIV PCR tests were negative, which by six months of age meant she had a 95 percent likelihood of being uninfected. Ms. X did not reveal her HIV status to anyone. Custody of Erica was shared between parents.

Ms. X continued to claim that she was not sexually active with Hubert. Appointments for Erica were scheduled in the family HIV clinic, which afforded Ms. X the opportunity to obtain her own medical care at the same time as Erica's appointments. Because of Ms. X's depressed CD4 count, her physician recommended she begin antiretroviral therapy and PCP prophylaxis. She declined this therapy and offers of help obtaining medication. It was thought that this was due, at least in part, to Ms. X not wanting these medicines around her house lest questions arise.

When Erica was ten months old, the social worker received a call from Erica's local pediatrician, informing her that he had just seen the child and was surprised to see Ms. X looking "very pregnant"—about five months according to Ms. X's own report. He advised her about an AZT therapy protocol that might greatly decrease the chances of the new baby becoming infected with HIV. Ms. X had not yet received prenatal care. The pediatrician informed her he would be contacting the social worker to help her arrange prenatal care (PNC). Ms. X informed him that Hubert was the father and that he was not aware of her HIV status.

The social worker contacted Ms. X to arrange PNC and to discuss further the AZT protocol. Ms. X informed the social worker that she arranged her own PNC and did not require assistance. She would not reveal the name of her physician or clinic. The social worker told Ms. X that the PNC provider needed to know her HIV status and should communicate with the hospital and clinic doctors regarding the protocol. Ms. X hung up the phone. She did this again during a subsequent call.

The social worker had the physician call the patient, and she listened to some information about the AZT protocol and agreed to an appointment at the nearby women's hospital. This appointment was not kept, but Ms. X did come with Erica to a family-clinic appointment. There the patient's clinic doctor made another appointment at the women's hospital that was kept. She was given prescriptions for AZT, which were not filled.

Approximately one week later, Ms. X began to experience difficulty breathing. She drove to a community hospital, did not reveal her HIV status to doctors there, but was transferred to the women's hospital due to her advanced pregnancy. At the women's hospital she also did not reveal her HIV status. She was admitted to the intensive care unit (ICU). Hospital staff located her prenatal chart (from the one PNC visit), and it revealed her HIV status. A diagnosis of PCP was made and patient was put on a ventilator.

Hubert and his family were beside themselves with anxiety. They remained in the ICU waiting room for days. They were told that Ms. X's condition was quite grave, and she might not make it. Hubert and his family were very angry that they weren't being given enough information about what was wrong with Ms. X. Meanwhile, the doctors, nurses, and social workers at the women's hospital were pleading with Ms. X to rectify this situation and inform Hubert of the nature of her illness. She refused these entreaties.

THE LANGUAGE AND ISSUES OF THE CASE

At several points in this case, two of the "classic" issues of the AIDS pandemic present themselves: (a) the issue whether there is a duty to warn sexual contacts of HIV-infected patients and (b) the question of whether treatment of pregnant women can in any sense be compelled, on the grounds of a duty to a fetus that she plans to carry to term. (This second issue is more explicitly debated in the literature on drug abuse and pregnancy.) Of great interest is that neither of those issues brought this case to a head. As in the previous case, the most important reason the treatment team desires to break confidentiality is simply out of concern for the patient-family relationship.

PERSPECTIVES AND KEY POINTS OF VIEW

Ms. X: She seems to be very concerned about what will happen to her relationship with Hubert if her HIV status is known to him. She fears that she will lose his affection and also that her economic and living situation will become very difficult without him. These fears are also intertwined with a variety of other issues such as a resentment that the health-care professionals are too involved in the intimate details of her life and that she has a right to her own privacy. But she is worried about what will happen should she and her children become very sick for a long time.

Hubert: He seems to "have been a saint" through all of this. He is concerned about Ms. X, Erica, and the baby she is about to deliver. But he is frustrated and confused. He is not sure whom to trust in all of this and is currently blaming the doctors for his lack of information. But at times he suspects that Ms. X is less than honest with him.

James: He seems to be reasonably dutiful toward Erica and her future. However, we know little about him, including whether he is HIV-infected, whether he is the source of Ms. X's HIV, and what he knows about his HIV status.

Caregivers: All of those intimately involved in the care of Ms. X and Erica have been "on the same page," since each has some prior experience in caring for patients with HIV. Although all would like Ms. X to be a model citizen who is fully adherent to her medical regimen and who is forthright with her sexual partners, the caregivers realize that they have to be careful not to alienate her. If they do, it was likely that Ms. X would seek still less medical care for herself and her children. But each caregiver was concerned that there had to be some line drawn at which they could not let the health and safety of others be further jeopardized. Nevertheless, they felt they first had to exhaust every possibility for forming a partnership with Ms. X.

WHAT ACTUALLY HAPPENED

Some days later, a decision was made to do an emergency C-section on Ms. X. Physicians informed Ms. X that unless she told Hubert about her diagnosis, they would. The baby would be discharged to Hubert, and he would need to administer both the AZT and the Bacitrim. Ms. X agreed to tell him after delivery. Ms. X followed through on this, informing Hubert that she had "just learned" she had AIDS. Hubert told his family, and all were extremely concerned, upset but quite caring and supportive of Ms. X.

The baby, Hubert Jr., did very well and was discharged to his father and his paternal grandparents. Hubert, the father, moved into his parents' home and everyone shared in the care of the baby. Everyone was informed about risks to the infant, and they were awaiting his first PCR test at age four weeks. Hubert's whole family continued to visit Ms. X, who was in the ICU after delivery of the baby.

James also visited Ms. X, although he had not been informed about her HIV status. While Ms. X was in the hospital, Erica had gone to stay with James and his parents. James's mother, however, was very suspicious and called the children's hospital's physician to inquire about whether her granddaughter Erica (now one year old) had ever been tested for HIV. She did not get a clear reply.

After weeks in the hospital, Ms. X was discharged, and Hubert's family agreed to take care of her in their home. (Erica remained with James and his parents.) Hubert Sr. was still quite devoted to Ms. X and vowed to stick by her. Very quickly, however, the situation deteriorated. Ms. X showed little interest in the baby, and Hubert's parents began to ask questions: Why was Erica going to the same doctors at the children's hospital that her half-brother Hubert Jr. had been seeing? What exactly was Erica being followed for at this hospital? And soon: When did Ms. X first learn of her HIV infection? Hubert's family did not get any direct answers from either Ms. X or the doctors and social workers. But they quickly began to feel they had been duped by Ms. X.

Ms. X was encouraged by the social worker to "come clean" with Hubert's family as her only hope of possibly saving her relationship with them. The social worker agreed to vouch that Ms. X was in "total denial" about her diagnosis and just could not deal with it. Ms. X agreed to think about this.

About one week later, Hubert's parents brought Hubert Jr. to the children's hospital. They mentioned that they had asked Ms. X to leave their home because she would not answer their questions, and they had to assume she had been horribly dishonest with them for too long. They were allowing her to live in the apartment she had previously shared with Hubert Sr. (which they owned), but were giving her a few weeks only, and she had a deadline to move out.

Ms. X at this point revealed her diagnosis to her mother, who resides in another state. James, the father of Erica, and his parents also learned of Ms. X's HIV but it is not clear who informed them. James subsequently had a negative HIV test. Hubert Sr. also tested negative, and Hubert Jr. has also had a negative PCR—making it very likely that he will have escaped HIV infection.

Ms. X had no further contact with Hubert Jr. although Hubert's parents had agreed to let her visit the baby "as long as they were home." She never called or arranged any visits. She did attempt to see Erica, but the paternal grandparents, who had been caring for her since Ms. X went into the hospital to have Hubert Jr. also insisted on a supervised visit.

The social worker helped Ms. X find an attorney to assist her with custody issues. A family court hearing was arranged regarding both children. Ms. X informed her attorney she did not want to get custody of Hubert Jr. and that she was comfortable having Hubert Sr. and his parents raise the baby. However, Ms. X did want shared custody of her one-year-old daughter. As she was living temporarily with a friend and had no home of her own, she was willing to accept an every-other-weekend custody arrangement. This was discussed between Ms. X and her attorney the day before her court hearing. Ms. X finished their conversation by adding that she would be coming to court with her new boyfriend and asked her attorney to make certain that HIV/AIDS did not come up in front of the boyfriend.

Although both James and Hubert Sr. were present at the hearing, and saw Ms. X in the company of her new boyfriend, the boyfriend was not told of any HIV issues.

COMMENTARY

Cases like this are usually seen as ones that pit the duties of the health-care provider to the patient against more general duties to keep others safe. And such cases ultimately may be reduced to that conflict of duties. However, the health-care team is to be commended for not immediately reducing this case to such a dilemma. They try to fulfill their duties to each of these parties by attempting to develop a fruitful relationship with Ms. X. If they can convince her that adherence to a plan of good medical treatment and that honesty with sexual partners is the best policy, everyone's interests will be served. Although they make some progress in this direction, things do not proceed quickly enough to head off the current conundrum.

Two points deserve noting:

1. The more clear and present the danger is to a third party, the greater the duty of the health-care providers to take steps to assist that person. One can argue that Hubert was a person clearly in such danger. But there are also obvious counterarguments available, especially before it became clear that he and Ms. X were having a sexual relationship. What the health-care providers should have done to protect Hubert seems to be a judgment call, and it is hard to criticize the caregivers up to this point.

2. Unlike an adult male, a fetus has no way to protect itself from possible infection. Therefore, the duty of the health-care team to aid this "patient" is probably clearer. (The question of whether a fetus is a person is moot; that Ms. X intends to deliver the baby means that the fetus will become a person even if it is not so earlier on.) However, as we saw in the case narrative, the con-

straints on this duty are largely practical but very formidable, e.g., sending the police to Ms. X's door may cause her to avoid treatment rather than seek it.

What we see in this case is that ethical duties are not absolute but are more-or-less affairs. It is also clear that as more and more alternatives are exhausted, as the danger to Hubert becomes more obvious, when the child is born and has its own independent medical needs, the duties to these third parties become stronger, and the duty to respect the patient's confidentiality loosens.

FOR FURTHER READING

Ronald Bayer, 1995. "Women's rights, babies' interests: Ethics, politics, and science in the debate of newborn HIV screening." In H. L. Minkoff, J. A. DeHovitz, A. Duerr, eds. *HIV infection in women*. New York, NY: Raven Press, 293–307.

James F. Childress, 1997. *Practical reasoning in bioethics*. Bloomington, IN: Indiana University Press, 95–118.

Lawrence O. Gostin, Zita Lazzarini, 1997. *Human rights and public health in the AIDS pandemic*. New York, NY: Oxford University Press.

Winifred J. Pinch, Charles J. Dougherty, V. McCarthy, 1995. "Ethics in nursing practice: Confidentiality for women and their children with HIV/AIDS." *Medsurg Nursing* 4(6): 452–57.

Arthur I. Segal, James A. Macer, S. Gainer Pillsbury, Russell Laros, George F. Lee, Tawfik Rizkallah, 1996. "Physician attitudes toward human immunodeficiency virus testing in pregnancy." *American Journal of Obstetrics and Gynecology* 174(6): 1750–56.

Morton Winston, Sheldon H. Landesman, 1987. Commentaries on Case Study, "AIDS and a duty to protect." *Hastings Center Report* 17(1): 2–23.

APPENDIX

Teaching Case Presentations: Materials to Assist You[1]

WHY WERE THESE MATERIALS WRITTEN AND HOW CAN THEY HELP?

In our clinical and continuing educational endeavors, we have asked medical students and health-care professionals to select and present cases they have encountered. The "hand-out" materials that follow have been designed for these two audiences. We found that these two groups have somewhat different needs. Medical students typically have a difficult time identifying relevant cases for presentation and are often not sure what information to bring to a case conference. Thus, we developed the Guidelines for Preparing Ethics Case Presentations that follow. It was geared to helping students to be complete in bringing out the necessary medical facts and thus making intelligent discussion possible. This factual emphasis is necessary because we found that medical students tend to fail in providing all relevant medical and social factors in favor of relating the case in terms of a conflict of values.

The key features of the Guidelines for Preparing Ethics Case Presentations are as follows. We attempt to circumscribe what may count as a suitable case for an ethics presentation. In this regard, we acknowledge that interpersonal conflict is usually the most obvious sign of an ethical issue at stake, but also suggest to the student that any case may serve this purpose as long as he or she provides all relevant information (e.g., the what, who, how, and why) of the decision-making process. We emphasize that three main items must be explored: the medical basis for decisions, the values being explicitly or implicitly promoted by each party to the decision-making process, and the com-

---

1. For additional information, see Mark Kuczewski, Mark R. Wicclair, Robert M. Arnold, Rosa Lynn Pinkus, Gretchen M. E. Aumann, 1994. "Make My Case: Ethics Teaching and Case Presentations." *Journal of Clinical Ethics* 5(4): 310–15

munication strategies that might have avoided problems in the process or that might now serve to alleviate further problems. Hence, we believe that the goal of case discussion is to lead the student from an understanding of the facts of the case to the values involved, but that the facts cannot be bypassed without severely distorting the discussion of the values at stake.

Because these guidelines were designed to help medical students who were presenting a case for discussion, they do not emphasize uncovering the perspectives of the parties to the case and the ethical issues and principles involved. If the student brings the facts to the conference, discussion can explore these dimensions.

Once the first draft of the cases that make up this book were submitted and reviewed by us, it was clear that the needs of health-care professionals were very different from those of the medical students. We found that medical professionals often provided detailed facts in their presentations but were more reluctant to speculate on the perspectives of the persons involved or their underlying values. We have only hypotheses as to the cause of this situation, but these tendencies seem to fit with professional experience and training.

Speculating on the perspectives of others is foreign and may even seem like "gossip" to the seasoned professional. Furthermore, the reluctance to make a recommendation to resolve the case could result from feeling they did not yet have the requisite expertise to make ethics recommendations or from fear of being "wrong," a fear that can be much more dreadful to one who is an expert than to a mere student. Also, a certain suspicion can cloud the working relationships in ethics discussions involving professionals. The stigma of the ethicist as a "moral cop" who is there to tell them what to do in their practices can cause the participants to be reluctant to use their moral imagination. It is just this speculative imagination that is needed to provide empathetic insight into the values and reasoning of the parties involved and to find creative resolutions to the problems at hand.

Thus, the pedagogical task was quite different with this group than it was in dealing with medical students. Rather than teach them to identify appropriate cases and report the facts, we needed to provide these professionals with a device that liberated their creativity and empathy. The task was to aid them in seeing how the patient's medical history, the perspectives of the parties to the decisions, and their future expectations are all rolled into one in the ethical dimension of a case. Thus, the concept of narrative was the idea chosen to help them give depth to their cases and provide descriptions that would be fruitful for others to explore in their teaching endeavors. This method of narrative presentation also provides them with a pedagogical device for imaginatively filling in facts, perspectives, and values as needed to guide their future casebook teaching sessions, where they will be dealing with cases for which they possess no real-life familiarity. Thus, the Guidelines for Written Case Presentation (Supplement 1): Narrative Presentation were drafted to make these ideas clear.

Guidelines for Preparing Ethics Case Presentations

WHAT CONSTITUTES AN ETHICS CASE OR ISSUE?

Students often select cases in which there is a conflict of opinion regarding the best course of action or treatment to pursue. Such conflicts can arise between physicians and patients, among members of the health-care team, between physicians and family members, between patients and family members, and among family members. Conflicts of this type can often be analyzed by focusing on the competing values of each party (e.g., extending life versus minimizing suffering). Presentations of cases involving conflicts can lead to discussions of such ethical issues as autonomy, competence (decision-making capacity), informed consent, paternalism, and the rights and responsibilities of physicians, patients, and family members.

Cases can be presented which do not involve any interpersonal conflicts. Students may wish to present a case because they believe that a decision was incompatible with an important ethical norm, value, or principle. For example, decision makers who seek to promote a patient's best interests (as perceived by the physician and family) may neglect the patient's right to information regarding the diagnosis, prognosis, and treatment alternatives. Thus, even though a physician and a patient's family may agree that the patient will not be told that she has cancer, the decision to withhold information may merit ethical examination.

Almost any case contains ethical issues because the norms of the doctor-patient relationship are ideally based on ethical principles and motivations. To identify ethical issues, students can select a case and observe how the physician-patient relationship is conducted. Particular attention can be given to how the attending and house staff interact with the patient, what and how information is conveyed, how and by whom treatment decisions are made, and how the patient's decision-making capacity is assessed. If a surrogate decision maker is involved, students might consider the following questions: How and by whom was it decided that the patient lacked decision-making capacity? How was the surrogate selected? Was sufficient information given to the surrogate? Was sufficient consideration given to the patient's values and best interests in the decision-making process?

Students are encouraged to discuss the decision-making process with the attending, house staff, and the patient or family. Such cases can facilitate an exploration during ethics conferences of the proper role of each party in treatment decisions, effective methods of communication, and means to minimize conflicts through better communication.

WHAT INFORMATION SHOULD I PRESENT?

The student should attempt to present all relevant medical and social facts about the patient. Ethically sound decision making is based on good medical care and a good factual basis regarding patient care. Much relevant information is easily obtainable from the patient's chart.

Students should attempt to understand the reasons and preferences of the parties involved. Doing so can help to identify important conflicts and their sources. On the other hand, seemingly unresolvable conflicts can be resolved when a sincere effort is made to understand the underlying reasons and values.

When preparing a case for presentation, the following questions may prove helpful:

1. Why does this case raise an ethical issue?
2. What values are being promoted/advanced in the patient's care?
3. Are there alternative values which are being neglected or thwarted?

What are the goals of the discussion?

1. To identify the ethical issues that arise in clinical medicine.
2. To help students develop the analytical tools needed to analyze difficult ethical problems and find justifiable solutions to those problems.
3. To enable students to recognize the kinds of cases that are likely to involve special ethical considerations and to develop justi-

fied strategies for addressing ethical concerns and preventing ethical conflicts.

4. To develop communication strategies and explore institutional strategies to arrive at more humane and ethical decisions.

Guidelines for Preparing an Ethics Case Presentation (Supplement 1) "Narrative Presentation"

(Especially for Use in *Written* Case Presentations)

WHAT IS NARRATIVE PRESENTATION OF A CASE?

Saying that cases in clinical medical ethics should be presented in narrative form is a fancy way of saying that we need to explain the case in ordinary language and try to convey its storylike quality. Presenting the case narratively is an attempt to trace and demonstrate the development of the themes that run through the case and that characterize the conflicts involved.

Narrating the case is much like what we do if we need to explain the case to a lay person. It is what we did all our lives before becoming health-care professionals. That is, we expressed things in ordinary language, usually beginning at some relevant point ("the beginning") and telling of the important events at each stage ("the action") until a pinnacle in the story is reached ("the climax"). The pinnacle is usually the height of the conflict between the main "characters" or the point at which one of the characters (e.g., the physician) faces a dilemma. This climax is usually what occasions us to present a case for discussion. We want to know how to resolve the conflict and help the characters achieve an ethically acceptable "resolution" (the final stage of the story).

WHY IS NARRATIVE FORM IMPORTANT?

On the one hand, there are mundane reasons for preferring a narrative account to a chart of "facts" concerning the case. For instance, narrating the case tends to make it more approachable to the nonspecialist or nonprofessional. Specialists in various medical fields often have their own jargon and abbreviations that are not readily accessible to other medical specialists, and health-care professionals must increasingly include lay persons in the decision-making and review process (e.g., the patient, the patient's family, medical ethics consultants, ethics committee members, etc.). Obviously, the more approachable format makes the case more usable by this wider variety of persons.

Of greater philosophical import is the notion that "facts" need to be interpreted, and narrative form is the easiest way of including the reader in that process. For example, large numbers of tests are often run on patients. Simply reporting the results of all tests will frequently not give the reader insight into which test results the health-care team is viewing as relevant or what conclusions they are drawing from them. Thus, the reasoning of the health-care professionals from the "facts" is hidden from us without a narrative account that thematizes the thought process.

Further, the health-care institution can be viewed as the junction of many "stories." The first or primary story is usually told from the perspective of the health-care team. It begins with the presentation of the patient for treatment and includes whatever information concerning the patient's medical history is available. This story features a climax and resolution in which the antagonist is the illness. This antagonist is overcome by or triumphs over the patient and the health-care team. In this story, the health-care team aids the protagonist (the patient) by helping him/her against the illness ("beneficence").

From the patient's perspective, the illness and the current presentation at the hospital are usually seen as one episode in the larger story of his or her life. This life includes dreams and goals, various significant relationships, beliefs and values, and a medical history that must be interpreted within the framework of this larger context, i.e., the patient's life. Within this context, an illness may not be the enemy simpliciter (in and of itself), to be defeated at all costs. For instance, a patient might authorize treatments because they offer hope of a cure but might decline these same treatments if he finds that they preclude a present quality of life that allows for certain highly valued daily activities. Further, the patient's sense of the "dignity" that characterizes his or her life is quite varied from one story to another. Thus, when the health-care team treats a patient only from the perspective of the primary narrative, the same actions may be valued differently in the patient's story. For example, what is beneficence in the primary narrative may be paternalism from the patient's perspective.

In sum, narrating the case allows us to make sense of it as if it were a novel. Simply reporting the "facts" often leaves us with the sense that characters are performing inexplicable or seemingly irrational acts for which the motivations are concealed. Narrative provides us with the motivations and reasoning of the health-care workers and helps us to find our first clues to the larger narrative that accounts for the actions and decisions of the patient. Once we frame the conflict within these larger stories, we often find that resolution is a matter of improved communication.

WHAT POINTS SHOULD I KEEP IN MIND TO IMPROVE MY CASE NARRATIVE?

There is no simple formula to make us perfect narrators of cases in clinical ethics any more than there is a rulebook that can make us novelists. However, just as there are conventions of writing fiction, there are some guidelines we should attempt to observe in writing case reports. For instance:

1. Medical jargon and abbreviations can be employed for terms frequently used. But translations clear to lay persons should be provided as well, usually parenthetically. However, jargon should never be used simply for its own sake even if you provide translations.
2. Most case presentations begin the story with the patient presenting for treatment. Keep in mind the larger narrative of the patient's life and try to include as much of the patient's larger history as is available to those health-care workers initially treating the patient. In other words, make sure you tell us what the treating physician knew about the patient at the time of the initial contact. This larger story often continues to be incrementally revealed to the health-care team. Include as much of this process of discovery in your report as is available.
3. Try to include the conclusions that the health-care professionals are drawing from their diagnostic work and tell how much of this information is conveyed to the patient. This is very important, because the two stories may be developing independently and may be based upon different information and conclusions.
4. No story is complete without an end. At various points in every story, the characters base their actions on what they believe will be the outcome. Medicine calls this outcome the prognosis. Surprisingly, this is often omitted from case reports. This happens because health-care workers often try to act as if they are dealing only with the empirical situation present at hand and

not venturing into future probabilities. However, in real life, we usually base our actions to some degree on our expectations of the future. This is true in both the medical narrative and the patient's life story. Hence, it is important to understand as much about the prognoses at the decision-making points as we can and to know how much of that information was conveyed to the patient/family.

5. Often, conflicts seem unresolvable at first glance. We look at the choices expressed by each party, and it seems that they cannot be reconciled. Often the choice of one of the parties seems irrational and unreasonable. In such cases we must ask why they are making the choice they are. There are many possible motivations for a decision, but motivations often can be traced to the larger narrative context of the patient's life. Asking the person directly why they have made the choice they have is always the preferred course of action. However, sometimes that is not possible. Attempt to provide as much of the patient's history as you deem may be relevant to understanding their motivations.

FOR FURTHER READING

Gretchen M. E. Aumann, Thomas R. Cole, 1991. "In whose voice? Composing a lifesong collaboratively." *Journal of Clinical Ethics* 2: 45–49.

Tod Chambers, 1996. "From the ethicist's point of view: The literary nature of ethical inquiry." *Hastings Center Report* 26(1): 25–32.

Rita Charon, 1994. "Narrative contributions to medical ethics: Recognition, formulation, interpretation, and validation in the practice of the ethicist." In E. R. Dubose, R. Hamel, L. J. O'Connell, eds. *A matter of principles? Ferment in U.S. bioethics*, Valley Forge, PA: Trinity Press International, 260–83.

Kathryn Montgomery Hunter, 1991. *Doctors' stories: The narrative structure of medical knowledge*. Princeton, NJ: Princeton University Press.

———1996. "Narrative, literature, and the clinical exercise of practical reason." *Journal of Medicine and Philosophy* 21(3): 303–20.

Mark Kuczewski, Mark R. Wicclair, Robert M. Arnold, Rosa Lynn Pinkus, Gretchen M. E. Aumann, 1994. "Make my case: Ethics teaching and case presentations." *Journal of Clinical Ethics* 5(4): 310–15.

Alasdair MacIntyre, 1984. *After virtue* (2nd ed.). Notre Dame: University of Notre Dame Press, see pp. 204–25.

Hilde Lindemann Nelson, 1997. *Stories and their limits: Narrative approaches to bioethics*. New York, NY: Routledge.

Daniel A. Putnam, 1988. "Virtue and the practice of modern medicine." *Journal of Medicine and Philosophy* 13(4): 433–43.

Works Cited

Agency for Health Care Policy and Research, 1993. *Depression in primary care.* Vol. 1, *Detection and diagnosis.* Rockville, MD: Public Health Service, U.S. Department of Health and Human Services, AHCPR Pub. No 93-0550.

Appelbaum, P. S. 1993. "Must we forgo informed consent to control health care costs? A response to Mark A. Hall." *Milbank Memorial Fund Quarterly* 71(4): 669–77.

Arras, J. D., ed. 1995. *Bringing the hospital home: Ethical and social implications of high-tech home care.* Baltimore, MD: The Johns Hopkins University Press.

Aumann, G. M. E., T. R. Cole. 1991. "In whose voice? Composing a lifesong collaboratively." *Journal of Clinical Ethics* 2: 45–49.

Bayer, R. 1995. "Women's rights, babies' interests: Ethics, politics, and science in the debate of newborn HIV screening." In H. L. Minkoff, J. A. DeHovitz, A. Duerr, eds. *HIV Infection in women.* New York, NY: Raven Press, pp. 293–307.

———1996a. "AIDS prevention—sexual ethics and responsibility." *New England Journal of Medicine* 334(23): 1540–42.

———1996b. "When victims need to know: Sometimes it's O.K. to test the accused for HIV." *New York Times*: Jan 18, A23.

Benton, E. C. 1990. "The constitutionality of pregnancy clauses in living will statutes." *Vanderbilt Law Review* 43(6): 1821–37.

Barendregt, J. J., L. Bonneux, and P. J. van der Maas, 1997. "The health care costs of smoking." *New England Journal of Medicine* 337(15): 1052–57.

Bernat, J. L., B. Gert, and R. P. Mogielnicky, 1993. "Patient refusal of hydration and nutrition: An alternative to physician-assisted suicide or voluntary active euthanasia." *Archives of Internal Medicine* 153: 2723–28.

Blackhall, L. J. 1987. "Must we always use CPR?" *New England Journal of Medicine* 317(20): 1281–85.

Blank, L. L. 1995. "Defining and evaluating physician competence in end-of-life patient care: A matter of awareness and emphasis." *Western Journal of Medicine* 163(3): 297–301.

Blustein, J. "The family in medical decisionmaking." *Hastings Center Report* 23(3): 6–13.

Bok, S. 1978. *Lying: Moral choice in public and private life.* New York: Pantheon Books.

Bradley, E., L. Walker, B. Blechner, T. Wetle, 1997. "Assessing capacity to participate in discussions of advance directives in nursing homes: Findings from a study of the patient self-determination act." *Journal of the American Geriatrics Society* 45(1): 79–83.

Brock, D. W. 1996. "What is the moral authority of family members to act as surrogates for incompetent patients?" *Milbank Memorial Fund Quarterly* 74(4): 599–618.

Brody, H. 1989. "Transparency: Informed consent in primary care." *Hastings Center Report* 19(5): 5–9.

Buchanan, A. E., and D. W. Brock, 1986. "Deciding for others." *Milbank Memorial Fund Quarterly* 64(2): 17–94.

———1989. *Deciding for others: The ethics of surrogate decision making*. New York: Cambridge University Press.

Burch, T. J. 1995. "Incubator or individual? The legal and policy deficiencies of pregnancy clauses in living will and advance health care directive statutes." *Maryland Law Review* 54(2): 528–70.

Callahan, D. 1992. "When self-determination runs amok." *Hastings Center Report* 22(2): 52–55.

Capezuti, E., L. Evans, N. Strumpf, and G. Maislin, 1996. "Physical restraint use and falls in nursing home residents." *Journal of the American Geriatric Society* 44(6): 627–33.

Caplan, A. L., D. Callahan, and J. Haas, 1987. "Ethical and policy issues in rehabilitation medicine." *Hastings Center Report* (Special Supplement) 17(4): S1–S19.

Chambers, T. 1996. "From the ethicist's point of view: The literary nature of ethical inquiry." *Hastings Center Report* 26(1): 25–32.

Charon, R. 1994. "Narrative contributions to medical ethics: Recognition, formulation, interpretation, and validation in the practice of the ethicist." In E. R. Dubose, R. Hamel, L. J. O'Connell, eds. *A matter of principles? Ferment in U.S. bioethics*. Valley Forge, PA: Trinity Press International, pp. 260–83.

Childress, J. F. 1997. *Practical reasoning in bioethics*. Bloomington, IN: Indiana University Press.

Churchill, L. R. 1987. *Rationing health care in America: Perceptions and principles of justice*. Notre Dame: University of Notre Dame Press.

———1989. "Trust, autonomy, and advance directives." *Journal of Religion and Health* 28(3): 175–83.

Clouser, K. D. 1977. "Allowing or causing: Another look." *Annals of Internal Medicine* 87(5): 622–24.

Council on Ethical and Judicial Affairs, American Medical Association, 1994. "Disputes between medical supervisors and trainees." *Journal of the American Medical Association* 272(23): 1861–65.

Davis, D. S. 1991. "Rich cases: The ethics of thick description." *Hastings Center Report* 21(4): 12–17.

Day, J., M. L. Smith, G. Erenberg, and R. L. Collins, 1994. "An assessment of a formal ethics committee consultation process." *HEC Forum* 6(1): 18–30.

Derse, A. R. 1990. "Ethics emergent." *Annals of Emergency Medicine* 19(2): 210–12.

DiNubile, M. J. 1990. "Responsibility for patient care: Where does the buck stop?" *American Journal of Medicine* 88(4): 405–406.

Downie, R. S., and F. Randall, 1997. "Parenting and the best interest of minors." *Journal of Medicine and Philosophy* 22(3): 219–31.

Drane, J. F. 1984. "Competency to give informed consent." *Journal of the American Medical Association* 252(7): 925–27.

————1985. "The many faces of competency." *Hastings Center Report* 15(2): 17–21.

Drickamer, M. A., M. A. Lee, and L. Ganzini, 1997. "Practical issues in physician–assisted suicide." *Annals of Internal Medicine* 126(2): 146–51.

Dworkin, R. 1993. *Life's dominion: An argument about abortion, euthanasia, and individual freedom.* New York: Alfred A. Knopf.

Emanuel, L. L. 1991. "The health care directive: Learning how to draft advance care documents." *Journal of the American Geriatric Society* 39(12): 1221–28.

Evans, L. K., N. E. Strumpf, 1989. "Tying down the elderly: A review of the literature on physical restraint." *Journal of the American Geriatric Society* 37(1): 65–74.

Evans, L. K., N. E. Strumpf, S. L. Allen-Taylor, E. Capezuti, G. Maislin, and B. Jacobsen, 1997. "A clinical trial to reduce restraints in nursing homes." *Journal of the American Geriatric Society* 45(6):675–81.

Faden, R. R., and T. L. Beauchamp, 1986. *A history and theory of informed consent.* New York: Oxford University Press.

Faden, R. R. 1997. "Managed care and informed consent." *Kennedy Institute of Ethics Journal* (7):377–79.

Ferrell, R. B., T. R. P. Price, B. Gert, and B. J. Bergen, 1984. "Volitional disability and physician attitudes toward noncompliance." *Journal of Medicine and Philosophy* 9(4): 333–52.

Finder, S. G. 1995. "Should competent patients or their families be able to refuse to allow an HEC case review? No." *HEC Forum* 7(1): 51–53.

Forrow, L., R. M. Arnold, and L. S. Parker, 1993. "Preventive ethics: Expanding the horizon of clinical ethics." *Journal of Clinical Ethics* 4(4): 287–94.

Forrow, L. 1994. "The green eggs and ham phenomena." *Hastings Center Report* 24(6): S29–S32.

Fox, R. C. 1980. "The evolution of medical uncertainty." *Milbank Memorial Fund Quarterly* 58(1): 1–49.

Frader, J. E. 1993. "Have we lost our senses? Problems with maintaining brain-dead bodies carrying fetuses." *Journal of Clinical Ethics* 4(4): 347–48.

Gervais, K. G., D. E. Vawter, and E. Spilseth, 1995. "Readings in rehabilitation ethics." *HEC Forum* 7(2): 183–97.

Gorlin, R., and H. D. Zucker, 1983. "Physicians' reactions to patients: A key to teaching humanistic medicine." *New England Journal of Medicine* 308(18): 1059–63.

Gostin, L. 1991. "The HIV-infected health care professional: Public policy, discrimination, and patient safety." *Archives of Internal Medicine* 151(4): 663–65.

————1997. "Health care information and the protection of personal privacy: Ethical and legal considerations." *Annals of Internal Medicine* 127(8, Pt.2): 683–90.

Gostin, L. O., and Z. Lazzarini, 1997. *Human rights and public health in the AIDS pandemic.* New York: Oxford University Press.

Greene, M. G., R. Adelman, R. Charon, and S. Hoffman, 1986. "Ageism in the medical encounter: An exploratory study of the doctor-elderly patient relationship." *Language and Communication* 6(½): 113–24.

Haas, J. 1993. "Ethical considerations of goal setting for patient care in rehabilitation medicine." *American Journal of Physical Medicine and Rehabilitation* 72(4): 228–32.

Hackler, J. C., and F. C. Hiller, 1990. "Family consent to orders not to resuscitate: Reconsidering hospital policy." *Journal of the American Medical Association* 264(10): 1281–83.

Hall, M. A. 1993. "Informed consent to rationing decisions." *Milbank Quarterly* 71(4): 645–67.

———1994. "Disclosing rationing decisions: A reply to Paul S. Appelbaum." *Milbank Quarterly* 72(2): 211–15.

Hardwig, J. 1990. "What about the family?" *Hastings Center Report* 20(2): 5–10.

Hill, C. S. 1993. "The barriers to adequate pain management with opioid analgesics." *Seminars in Oncology* 20(2): S1: 1–5.

Hunter, K. M. 1991. *Doctors' stories: The narrative structure of medical knowledge.* Princeton, NJ: Princeton University Press.

———1996. "Narrative, literature, and the clinical exercise of practical reason." *Journal of Medicine and Philosophy* 21(3): 303–20.

Iserson, K. V. 1995. "If we don't learn from history . . . : Ethical failings in a new prehospital directive." *American Journal of Emergency Medicine* 13(2): 241–42.

———1996. "Withholding and withdrawing medical treatment: An emergency medicine perspective." *Annals of Emergency Medicine* 28(1): 51–54.

Jonsen, A. R. 1991a. "Of balloons and bicycles, or The relationship between ethical theory and practical judgment." *Hastings Center Report* 21(5): 14–16.

———1991b. "Casuistry as a methodology in clinical ethics." *Theoretical Medicine* 12(4): 295–307.

Junkerman, C., and D. Schiedermayer, 1998. *Practical ethics for students, interns, and residents: A short reference manual,* 2nd ed. Frederick, MD: University Publishing Group. Original edition, 1994.

Kane, R. A., and A. L. Caplan, eds. 1993. *Ethical conflicts in the management of home care: The case manager's dilemma.* New York: Springer Publishing Company.

Kapp, M. B. 1992. "Nursing home restraints and legal liability: Merging the standard of care and industry practice." *Journal of Legal Medicine* 13(1): 1–32.

Kass, L. R. 1991. "Why doctors must not kill." *Commonweal* 118(14): 472–76.

Katz, J. 1984a. *The silent world of doctor and patient.* New York: Free Press.

———1984b. "Why doctors don't disclose uncertainty." *Hastings Center Report* 14(1): 35–44.

Kelly, D. F. 1991. *Critical care ethics: Treatment decisions in american hospitals.* Kansas City, MO: Sheed & Ward.

Kopelman, L. M. 1997. "The best-interests standard as threshold, ideal, and standard of reasonableness." *Journal of Medicine and Philosophy* 22(3): 271–89.

Kroeger-Mappes, J. 1996. "Ethical dilemmas for nurses: Physician's orders versus patient's rights." In T. A. Mappes, D. DeGrazia, eds. *Biomedical Ethics*, 4th ed. pp. 139–46.

Kuczewski, M., M. R. Wicclair, R. M. Arnold, R. L. Pinkus, G. M. E. Aumann, 1994. "Make my case: Ethics teaching and case presentations." *Journal of Clinical Ethics* 5(4): 310–15.

Kuczewski, M. G. 1996. "Reconceiving the family: The process of consent in medical decisionmaking." *Hastings Center Report* 26(2): 30–37.

———1997. *Fragmentation and consensus: Communitarian and casuist bioethics*. Washington, DC: Georgetown University Press.

———1998a. "Casuistry." In Ruth Chadwick, ed., *Encyclopedia of Applied Ethics*. San Diego: Academic Press, Vol. 1: 423–32.

———1998b. "Physician-assisted death: Can philosophical bioethics aid social policy?" *Cambridge Quarterly of Healthcare Ethics* 7(4): 339–47.

———1999. "Ethics in long-term care: Are the principles different?" *Theoretical Medicine and Bioethics* 20(1).

Lantos, J., and A. Kohrman, 1992. "Ethical aspects of pediatric home care." *Pediatrics* 89(5): 920–24.

Lantos, J.D. 1997. *Do we still need doctors?* New York: Routledge.

Lederman, A. D. 1994. "A womb of my own: A moral evaluation of Ohio's treatment of pregnant patients with living wills." *Case Western Reserve Law Review* 45(1): 351–77.

Lidz, C. W., A. Meisel, M. Osterweis, J. L. Holden, J. H. Marx, M. R. Munetz, 1983. "Barriers to informed consent." *Annals of Internal Medicine* 99(4): 539–43.

Lidz, C. W., P. S. Appelbaum, and A. Meisel, 1988. "Two models of implementing informed consent." *Archives of Internal Medicine*, 148: 185–89.

Lidz, C. W., L. Fischer, and R. M. Arnold, 1992. *The Erosion of Autonomy in Long-Term Care*. New York: Oxford University Press.

Lidz, C. W., and R. M. Arnold, 1993. "Rethinking autonomy in long-term care." *Miami Law Review* 47(3): 603–23.

Lurie, S. G. 1994. "Ethical dilemmas and professional roles in occupational medicine." *Social Science and Medicine* 38(10): 1367–74.

Lyness J. M., T. K. Noel, C. Cox, D. A. King, Y. Conwell, and E. D. Caine, 1997. "Screening for depression in elderly primary care patients: A comparison of the center for epidemiologic studies' depression scale and the geriatric depression scale." *Archives of Internal Medicine* 157(4): 449–54.

MacAvoy-Snitzer, J. 1987. "Pregnancy clauses in living will statutes." *Columbia Law Review* 87(6): 1280–1300.

MacIntyre, A. 1984. *After virtue*. 2nd ed. Notre Dame: University of Notre Dame Press.

Macklin, R. 1987. *Mortal choices*. Boston, MA: Houghton Mifflin Company.

McCrary, S. V., W. L. Allen, and C. L. Young, 1993. "Questionable competency of a surrogate decision maker under a durable power of attorney." *Journal of Clinical Ethics* 4(2): 166–68.

Mechanic, D. 1994. "Trust and informed consent to rationing." *Milbank Quarterly* 72(2): 217–23.

Meier, D. E., S. R. Morrison, and C. K. Cassel, 1997. "Improving palliative care." *Annals of Internal Medicine* 127(3): 225–30.

Meisel, A., A. Grenvik, R. L. Pinkus, and J. V. Snyder, 1986. "Hospital guidelines for deciding about life-sustaining treatment: Dealing with health limbo." *Critical Care Medicine* 14(3): 239–46.

Meisel, A. 1991. "Legal myths about terminating life support." *Archives of Internal Medicine* 151: 1497–1502.

————1992. "The legal consensus about forgoing life-sustaining treatment: Its status and prospects." *Kennedy Institute of Ethics Journal* 2(4): 309–45.

Meisel, A., and S. K. Dorst. 1992a. "Living wills given life in Pa." *Pennsylvania Law Journal* XV(29): 5,29.

————1992b. "Work in progress: Pa.'s living will law leaves unanswered question." *Pennsylvania Law Journal* XV(31): 5, 10, 23.

Meisel, A., and M. Kuczewski, 1996. "Legal and ethical myths about informed consent." *Archives of Internal Medicine* 156: 2521–26.

Miles, S. H., P.A. Singer, and M. Siegler, 1989. "Conflicts between patients' wishes to forgo treatment and the policies of health care facilities." *New England Journal of Medicine* 321(1): 48–50.

Miles, S. H. 1992. "Medical futility." *Law, Medicine & Health Care* 20(4): 310–15.

Miles, S. H., and R. Meyers, 1994. "Untying the elderly." *Clinics in Geriatric Medicine* 10(3): 513–25.

Miller, F. H. 1992. "Denial of health care and informed consent in English and American law." *American Journal of Law and Medicine* 18(1&2): 37–71.

Miller, F. G., and H. Brody, 1995. "Professional integrity and physician-assisted death." *Hastings Center Report* 25(3): 8–17.

Minogue, B., and J. E. Reagan, 1994. "Can complex legislation solve our end-of-life problems?" *Cambridge Quarterly of Healthcare Ethics* 3(1):115–24.

Morreim, E. H. 1989. "Fiscal scarcity and the inevitability of bedside budget balancing." *Archives of Internal Medicine* 149: 1012–15.

————1995. *Balancing act: The new medical ethics of medicine's new economics.* Washington, DC: Georgetown University Press.

Moss, A. H., and M. Siegler, 1991. "Should alcoholics compete equally for liver transplantation?" *Journal of the American Medical Association* 265(10): 1295–97.

Murphy, D. J. 1988. "Do-not-resuscitate orders: Time for reappraisal in long-term care institutions." *Journal of the American Medical Association* 260(14): 2098–2101.

Nash, D. B., L. E. Markson, S. Howell, and E. A. Hildreth, 1993. "Evaluating the competence of physicians in practice: From peer review to performance assessment." *Academic Medicine* 68(2 Suppl): S19–22.

National Citizens' Coalition for Nursing Home Reform, 1996. *Individualized care approaches to reduce the use of chemical and physical restraints.* Washington, DC: NCCNHR.

Nelson, J. L. 1992. "Taking families seriously." *Hastings Center Report* 22(4): 6–12.

————. 1997. *Stories and their limits: Narrative approaches to bioethics.* New York Routledge.

Nelson, H. L. and J. L. Nelson, 1995. *The patient in the family: An ethic of medicine and families*. New York: Routledge.

Noddings, N. 1995. "Moral obligation or moral support for high-tech home care?" In John D. Arras ed., *Bringing the hospital home: Ethical and social implications of high-tech home care*. Baltimore, MD: The Johns Hopkins University Press, pp. 149–65.

Novack, D., B. J. Detering, R. Arnold, L. Forrow, M. Ladinsky, and J. Pezzullo, 1989. "Physicians' attitudes toward using deception to resolve difficult ethical problems." *Journal of the American Medical Association* 261(20): 2980–85.

Passell, P., 1993. "Experts wavering on steep rise in cigarette tax," *New York Times*, June 7, A8.

Pear, R., 1993. "The disabled gain new rights to jobs and health insurance; 'Equal Access' ruling affects millions in U.S.," *New York Times*, June 9. A1 & A10.

Pearlman, R. A. 1993. "Forgoing medical nutrition and hydration: An area for fine-tuning skills." *Journal of General Internal Medicine* 8: 225–27.

Pence, G. E. 1995. *Classic cases in medical ethics*. 2nd ed. New York: McGraw-Hill.

Pinch, W. J., C. J. Dougherty, and V. McCarthy, 1995. "Ethics in nursing practice: Confidentiality for women and their children with HIV/AIDS." *MEDSURG Nursing* 4(6): 452–57.

Pinkus, R. L. B. 1996. "Politics, paternalism and the rise of the neurosurgeon: The evolution of moral reasoning." *Medical Humanities Review* 10(2): 20–44.

Portenoy, R. K. 1993. "Cancer pain management." *Seminars in Oncology* 20(2); S1: 19–35.

Povar, G. J. 1993. "Second guessing the patient's trust: Facing the challenge of the difficult surrogate." *Journal of Clinical Ethics* 4(2): 168–71.

President's commission for the study of ethical problems in medicine and biomedical and behavioral research, 1982. *Making health care decisions*, Vol. 1. Washington, DC: U.S. Government Printing Office.

———, 1983. *Deciding to forego life-sustaining treatment*. Washington, DC: U.S. Government Printing Office.

Purtilo, R. B. 1984. "Applying the principles of informed consent to patient care: Legal and ethical considerations for physical therapy." *Physical Therapy* 64: 934–37.

———. 1988. "Ethical issues in teamwork: The context of rehabilitation." *Archives of Physical Medicine and Rehabilitation* 69(5): 318–22.

Putnam, D. A. 1988. "Virtue and the practice of modern medicine." *Journal of Medicine and Philosophy* 13(4): 433–43.

Quill, T. E. 1991. "Death and dignity: A case of individualized decision making." *New England Journal of Medicine* 324(10): 691–94.

Quill, T. E., C. K. Cassel, and D. E. Meier, 1994. "Care of the hopelessly ill: Proposed clinical criteria for physician-assisted suicide." *New England Journal of Medicine* 327(19):1380–84.

Reiser, S. J. 1994. "The ethical life of health care organizations." *Hastings Center Report* 24(6): 28–35.

Roberts, L. W., T. McCarty, G. Thaler, 1995. "Should competent patients or their families be able to refuse to allow an HEC case review? Yes." *HEC Forum* 7(1): 48–50.

Rodwin, M. A. 1993. *Medicine, money & morals: Physicians' conflicts of interest.* New York: Oxford University Press.

Ross, J. W., C. Bayley, V. Michel, and D. Pugh, 1986. *Handbook for hospital ethics committees.* Chicago, IL: American Hospital Publishing.

Ross, J. W., J. Glaser, D. Rasinski-Gregory, J. M. Gibson, 1993. *Health care ethics committees. The next generation.* Chicago, IL: American Hospital Publishing.

Sabatino, C. P. 1993. "Surely the wizard will help us, Toto? Implementing the patient self-determination act." *Hastings Center Report* 23(1): 12–16.

Sachs, G. A., S. H. Miles, and R. A. Levin, 1991. "Limiting resuscitation: Emerging policy in emergency medical systems." *Annals of Internal Medicine* 114(2): 151–54.

Sachs, G. A., J. C. Ahronheim, J. A. Rhymes, L. Volicer, and J. Lynn, 1995. "Good care of dying patients: The alternative to physician-assisted suicide and euthanasia." *Journal of the American Geriatrics Society* 43: 553–62.

Schneiderman, L. J., N. S. Jecker, and A. R. Jonsen, 1990. "Medical futility: Its meaning and implications." *Annals of Internal Medicine* 112(12): 949–54.

Schneiderman, L. J., and N. S. Jecker, 1995. *Wrong medicine: Doctors, patients, and futile treatment.* Baltimore, MD: Johns Hopkins University Press.

Schnelle, J. F., P. G. MacRae, S. F. Simmons, G. Uman, J. G. Ouslander, L. L. Rosenquist, and B. Chang, 1994. "Safety assessment for frail elderly: A comparison of restrained and unrestrained nursing home residents." *Journal of the American Geriatric Society* 42(6): 586–92.

Scofield, G. R. 1995. "The problem of (non-)compliance: Is it patients or patience?" *HEC Forum* 7(2-3): 150–65.

Scott, R. A., L. H. Aiken, D. Mechanic, and J. Moravcsik, 1995. "Organizational aspects of caring." *Milbank Memorial Fund Quarterly* 73(1): 77–95.

Segal, A. I., J. A. Macer, S. G. Pillsbury, R. Laros, G. F. Lee, T. Rizkallah, 1996. "Physician attitudes toward human immunodeficiency virus testing in pregnancy." *American Journal of Obstetrics and Gynecology* 174(6): 1750–56.

Sheldon, M. 1982. "Truth telling in medicine." *Journal of the American Medical Association* 247(5): 651–54.

Shortell, S. M., R. R. Gillies, and K. J. Devers, 1995. "Reinventing the American hospital." *Milbank Memorial Fund Quarterly* 73(2): 131–60.

Shreves, J. G., and A. H. Moss, 1996. "Residents ethical disagreements with attending physicians: An unrecognized problem." *Academic Medicine* 71(10): 1103–1105.

Siegler, M. M. 1982. "Confidentiality in medicine: A decrepit concept." *New England Journal of Medicine* 307(24): 1518–21.

Silverman, H. J. 1994. "Revitalizing a hospital ethics committee." *HEC Forum* 6(4): 189–222.

Silverman, L. M., and M. Dennis; F. Rouse, and D. Smith, 1992. Commentaries on "Whether no means no." *Hastings Center Report* 22(2): 26–27.

Slomka, J. 1994. "The ethics committee: Providing education for itself and others." *HEC Forum* 6(1): 31–38.

Sosna, D. P., M. Christopher, M. M. Pesto, D. V. Morando, and J. Stoddard, 1994. "Implementation strategies for a do-not-resuscitate program in the prehospital setting." *Annals of Emergency Medicine* 23(5): 1042–46.

Stell, L. K. 1992. "Stopping treatment on grounds of futility: A role for institutional policy." *St. Louis University Public Law Review* 11: 481–97.

Stoeckle, J. D. 1995. "The citadel cannot hold: Technologies go outside the hospital, patients and doctors too." *Milbank Memorial Fund Quarterly* 73(1): 3–17.

Strong, C. 1984. "The neonatologist's duty to patient and parents." *Hastings Center Report* 14(4): 10–16.

Sullivan, M. D., and S. J. Youngner, 1994. "Depression, competence, and the right to refuse lifesaving medical treatment." *American Journal of Psychiatry* 15(1): 971–78.

Sullivan, R. J. 1993. "Accepting death without artificial nutrition or hydration." *Journal of General Internal Medicine* 8(4): 220–24.

Teno, J. and J. Lynn, 1991. "Voluntary active euthanasia: The individual case and public policy." *Journal of the American Geriatrics Society* 39: 827–30.

Tinetti, M. E., L. Wen-Liang, and S. R. Ginter, 1992. "Mechanical restraint use and fall-related injuries among residents of skilled nursing facilities." *Annals of Internal Medicine* 116(5):369–74.

Tomlinson, T., and H. Brody, 1988. "Ethics and communication in do-not-resuscitate orders." *New England Journal of Medicine* 318(1): 43–46.

———, 1990. "Futility and the ethics of resuscitation." *Journal of the American Medical Association* 264(10): 1276–80.

Tomlinson, T., and D. Czlonka, 1995. "Futility and hospital policy." *Hastings Center Report* 25(3): 28–35.

Toulmin, S.E. 1986. "Divided loyalties and ambiguous relationships." *Social Science and Medicine* 23(8): 783–87.

Truog, R. D., A. S. Brett, and J. Frader, 1992. "The problem with futility." *New England Journal of Medicine* 326(23): 1560–64.

Ubel, P. A., and R. M. Arnold, 1995. "The unbearable rightness of bedside rationing." *Archives of Internal Medicine* 155:1837–42.

Ubel, P. A., and S. Goold, 1997. "Bedside rationing: Clear cases and tough calls." *Annals of Internal Medicine* 126(1): 74–80.

Veatch, R. 1987. *Case studies in medical ethics*. Philadelphia, PA: Lippincott.

Waisel, D. B., and R. D. Truog, 1995. "The cardiopulmonary resuscitation-not-indicated order: Futility revisited." *Annals of Internal Medicine* 122(4): 304–308.

Walsh, D. C. 1986. "Divided loyalties in medicine: The ambivalence of occupational medical practice." *Social Science and Medicine* 23(8): 789–96.

Weissman, D. E. 1996. "Cancer pain education for physicians in practice: Establishing a new paradigm." *Journal of Pain and Symptom Management* 12(6): 364–71.

Werner, P., V. Koroknay, J. Braun, and J. Cohen-Mansfield, 1994. "Individualized care: alternatives used in the process of removing physical restraints in the nursing home." *Journal of the American Geriatric Society* 42(3): 321–25.

Wicclair, M. R. 1991. "Patient decision-making capacity and risk." *Bioethics* 5(2):91–104.

———. 1993. *Ethics and the elderly*, New York: Oxford University Press.

Winston, M.; S. H. Landesman, 1987. Commentaries on Case Study, "AIDS and a Duty to Protect." *Hastings Center Report* 17(1): 22–23.

Woodstock Theological Center, 1995. *Ethical considerations in the business aspects of health care.* Washington, DC: Georgetown University Press.

Youngner, S. J. 1987. "Do-not-resuscitate orders: No longer secret, but still a problem." *Hastings Center Report* 17(1): 24–33.

———1988. "Who defines futility?" *Journal of the American Medical Association* 260(14): 2094–95.

Name Index

Subject Index